HOSPICE CARE AND CULTURE

Hospice Care and Culture

A comparison of the Hospice Movement in the West and Japan

TERESA CHIKAKO MARUYAMA

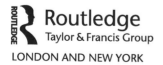

Taylor & Francis Group

LONDON AND NEW YORK

First published 1999 by Ashgate Publishing

Reissued 2018 by Routledge
2 Park Square, Milton Park, Abingdon, Oxon OX14 4RN
711 Third Avenue, New York, NY 10017, USA

Routledge is an imprint of the Taylor & Francis Group, an informa business

Publisher's Note
The publisher has gone to great lengths to ensure the quality of this reprint but points out that some imperfections in the original copies may be apparent.

Disclaimer
The publisher has made every effort to trace copyright holders and welcomes correspondence from those they have been unable to contact.

A Library of Congress record exists under LC control number: 98074201

ISBN 13: 978-1-138-31748-2 (hbk)
ISBN 13: 978-1-138-31927-1 (pbk)
ISBN 13: 978-0-429-45389-2 (ebk)

Contents

11 Conclusion 155

Acknowledgements

The study from which this book arises was carried out over four years while I was at the Centre for Philosophy and Health Care at the University of Wales, Swansea. Portions of it have previously been published as 'The Japanese Pilgrimage: Not Begun' in the *International Journal of Palliative Nursing* (Vol.3, No.2, March-April 1997, pp.87-91), and I would like to thank the publisher for permission to use them here. This study would not have been possible without help from countless people and it is a pity that I cannot mention all of their names. But I would like to record my special thanks to all the members of the staff and secretaries of the Centre, particularly my supervisor Dr David A. Greaves, who has always given me useful advice and been patiently supportive of my academic life, and Ms Louise de Raeve, who has made useful comments and pointed out good literature sources. My genuine thanks are also due to Fr Francis Mackenna and Mr Neil J. Pickering, who are my best friends in Britain and have given me a lot of psychological as well as spiritual support in my most difficult and lonely times. I must give my heartfelt thanks as well to the many cancer patients and those in bereavement who I met in hospices, hospitals and various other places here in Britain as well as in Japan over the past years, many of whom encouraged me to carry on this work, though sadly some of them have already died before its completion. I am also very grateful to Yvonne Saunders, a cleaning lady for our building, who has always considered my convenience so that I can use the coffee room until very late at night whenever I have to stay up late in the department.

Being resident in Britain for more than four years, I have made friends with many British people and others from all over the world from more than 20 countries who are studying at the university. This vivid experience of cross-cultural communication with various races has enabled me to make cultural comparisons not only in my academic work but also in my ordinary day-to-day life. Although this research has been a philosophical enquiry about the hospice movement comparing the West and Japan, this rich cultural experience has inspired me in writing this book. So I gratefully acknowledge these friends from throughout the world beginning with Britain. Finally, let me send my thanks to my family who have been understanding towards my study and always very supportive from afar.

1 Introduction

An expression like 'the West', which is used in the title and will be used throughout this book, can easily be attacked for its over generalization and simplification. There are many different cultures inside the Western world. It may also seem wrong to use the term 'the Western hospice movement', since there are some Western countries which have not yet established any institution named a 'hospice'. We would like to say, however, that it may be acceptable to use this phrase 'the Western hospice' in this study. Many Western countries have shared some general historical changes which have influenced the Western medical culture, for example, the doctor's status, medical science, and also the Western perspective on life and death in relation to Christianity, the rise of individualism and the Enlightenment. The important thing is to look at how this common background, tendency, and change amongst different Western countries will relate to the care of the dying, particularly terminal cancer patients in Japan, when Japan imports the Western hospice movement. On the other hand, we should not bring the term 'the East' as an object for comparison with the West, because our primary interest is to consider what will be the issues in applying the Western hospice movement especially to Japanese medicine. This requires us to explore the details of the Japanese situation in regard to the care of cancer patients, attitudes to death and dying, and the doctor-patient relationship, and to distinguish them from those of other Eastern countries.

Another important question we have to raise at the very beginning of the book is whether one can make a cultural comparison or can understand both the Western and the Japanese culture in an objective way. We are not sure if it is possible for the writer of this book, I myself, to understand both the Western and the Japanese cultures. To some extent, I have been deeply influenced by Western culture; have an English name, TERESA; have been given a Catholic education since my childhood (though in Japan), and have lived in Great Britain for more than four years while studying at the University of Wales, Swansea. The way I think, look at things, and behave, whether consciously or unconsciously, may appear westernized in other Japanese people's eyes.

1

On the other hand it may be also true that I have not been able completely to discard all my Japanese ways of thinking or behaving in only four years, because I have been brought up in a Japanese family and culture for the past twenty odd years. I may be acting, without awareness, in a very 'typical Japanese way' in Western people's eyes, and will be treated as a Japanese or an Easterner by them no matter how many more years I live in this country. Thus I may be neither purely Japanese nor Western (British for example) and that means I have written this book, to some extent, as a 'half outsider' of both the Japanese as well as the Western culture. So I may be able truly to appreciate neither of the two cultures.

There is always the temptation of extreme cultural relativism in making a comparison between two cultures, by drawing too clear a line between them. But the experience of a person like myself could be a kind of evidence that the West and Japan share some basic moral values and that they cannot be totally separable, otherwise, I would not have been able to live in the West for four years, and make any sense of the experience. If there was no continuity between the two cultures at all, I would have needed 'brainwashing' in order completely to destroy my moral values as a Japanese person and change them into absolutely new ones so that I could adjust to life in the West. It is unrealistic to imagine that such 'brainwashing', which could create a 'completely new identity', can be done within four years. There is therefore no such a thing as perfect cultural relativism which determines that different cultures are unable to share moral values at all and in which ethical issues become merely a matter of culture. It is not of primary interest here to discuss the philosophical question of the existence of a universal innate moral awareness of humans beyond cultural differences, but to clarify the position taken in this study before going on to the main chapters so that we do not attempt to look at the two cultures as black-and-white. I may be a 'half outsider' but that means I am also a 'half insider' of the two cultures, and this may give me a positive advantage in getting a picture of both cultures and prevent the 'temptation' of extreme cultural relativism.

However, we will nevertheless discover some significant differences and difficulties in bringing the Western hospice philosophy to the Japanese medical culture. The main aim of this study is not to give any simple answer to these issues, but to determine some of the crucial questions that need to be considered, which have not yet been analyzed sufficiently in Japanese medicine. There will be no proper answers unless we find the right questions.

PART I
THE HOSPICE MOVEMENT
IN THE WEST AND IN
JAPAN

2 The Hospice Movement in the West

Introduction

It has become understood that hospice care is/will be one of the important alternative ways for the care of the terminally ill, especially, cancer patients. In this chapter, let us consider the nature of the Western hospice movement from several aspects, which will be a helpful basis for chapter 5, where we analyze how an attitude to death and dying and the doctor-patient relationship are reflected in the care of cancer patients in the West. We will tend to discuss the British hospice movement, since the modern hospice has its origin in Britain, and has more or less influence on hospices throughout the world, and we can see clearly and interestingly the crucial nature and underlying notions of the hospice there.

The History of the Hospice

First of all, let us consider how the term 'hospice' was born in the West and how it became a place particularly for cancer patients in the modern period. This historical analysis is necessary in order to understand the current problems raised by the modern hospice movement in the West, because such study reveals the process by which they have been created.

The Origin of the Word 'Hospice'

The word 'hospice' came from the Latin 'hospes' which meant 'guest' but by late classical times, under the influence of Christianity, had changed to mean 'a stranger' not known personally to the host (Talbot, 1967, p.386; cited by Manning, 1984, p.33). Cicero (116-43 BC) said that 'hospes' implies a 'host' who welcomed an unexpected visitor and that 'hospitalis' meant 'friendly'. A similar word for 'hospitium' in the Greek language was 'xenodochion' translated as a 'place to receive the stranger', in which 'xenos' meant 'stranger'. In the Greek Bible, the term 'xenos' is used: 'I was a stranger (xenos) and ye took me in' (Matthew 25: 35).

Jesus actually intended to say that we have to find Jesus (God) within each strange visitor, and to treat strangers lovingly as we do God. So 'hospitium' or pilgrims and strangers are called 'xenodochia'. It is important to notice that in the classical era there was no idea of 'the dying' nor 'cancer patients', whether Latin or Greek, in relation to the term 'hospice', and the reason why 'guest' or 'stranger' has become replaced by 'the dying' or 'cancer patients' between the medieval and the modern age should be considered as one of the serious problems in the modern hospice movement, which we will discuss later in Section 3 (Manning, 1984, pp.33-34).

The Distinction between 'Hospital' and 'Hospice' in Medieval Times

There was no clear distinction between 'hospice' and 'hospital' in medieval times.   The Latin word for 'hospital' is 'hospitale' or 'hospitalia'.   The former means 'a large house, or place' and the latter, 'apartments for strangers', which reminds us readily of the original concept of the word 'hospice' (*An Etymological Dictionary of the English Language*, p.272).   Presumably, however, a 'hospital' tends to be bigger in scale than a 'hospice' as the Latin word 'hospitale' or 'hospitalia' implies 'a large house'.   Carlin tries to identify 'hospice' with one of the four classifications of hospital in the medieval period: 'leper houses, almshouses, hospices for poor wayfayers and pilgrims, and institutions that cared for the sick poor'.   None of the four supplied any professional medical care as modern hospitals do today.   The inmates in leper houses and almshouses led 'a semi-monastic life'.   The fourth class identified by Carlin was uncommon and mainly cared for the non-leprous sick and poor (Carlin, 1989, pp.21-24).   Taking the other three kinds of hospitals into consideration, let us now look at the more detailed history of the 'hospital' called a 'hospice' in Carlin's third class.

The Emergence of the Distinction between 'Hospital' and 'Hospice'

In the West, the hospice called a 'hospitium' already existed in Rome from the seventh or the eighth century, as a shelter for pilgrims visiting the tomb of St Peter.   There was no evidence that the 'hospitium' gave any medical treatment except simply giving first aid for cuts and travel sores, nor that it was a place for the sick or the dying (Talbot, 1967; cited by Manning 1984, p.34).   In the Middle Ages, the hospice flourished in Europe, and one of the typical hospices was located in Jerusalem, founded in 1100 AD by Brother Gerald, a member of the Knights Hospitallers of St John. The knights hospitallers expanded and established similar hospices in Italy, Germany, Malta, and England. The philosophy of these early hospices regarded the care of the soul to be as important as that of the body, so faith and love were considered to be more necessary than skill and science in the medieval hospice. Different religious foundations from the earliest times sheltered all comers especially Christian travellers and pilgrims and named themselves 'hospices' (Manning, 1984, pp.34-38).

At that time it was not easy to draw a line between a 'hospice' and the other three kinds of hospitals, where no professional medical care was given and the treatment of the inmate was care-centred. However it might be possible to say that hospices took a bigger part in caring for travellers and pilgrims than other hospitals did, though there seemed only a limited number of hospices dealing solely with people of this sort. Although the modern hospice movement emphasizes care-centred treatment for the dying, which challenges the modern hospitals' cure-centred way, it was not necessary for the medieval hospice to be against the other three kinds of hospitals, since all of them were care-centred as much as the hospice was, and all lacked medical knowledge and facilities at that time. How have the ideas of hospice and hospital then come almost to oppose each other as the centuries have passed? To answer the question we need to see how the 'hospice-like hospital' in medieval times has been transformed into today's hospital. Let us look at the process of the medicalization of medieval hospitals next.

The medicalization of hospitals began after the Black Death that occurred in the middle of the fourteenth century and 'led to the immediate diversion of all charitable funds to medical hospitals' (Henderson, 1989, p.70). As we will discuss in a later chapter on the history of the Western doctor's status, however, it might be that the rise of the secular medical profession had already begun in the twelfth century. Before then, hospitals were under the order of the church, but from the twelfth century church councils forbade monks to go out from the monastery to give medical treatments to people outside so that monks would concentrate more on their religious work. This prohibition became the foundation of building secular medical schools and was the beginning of the separation of the medical profession from the church. Therefore, this change in the twelfth century should be considered as an important background against which the real medicalization arose from the time of the Black Death.

A real transformation of the hospitals from a 'general refuge' into a place only for the sick, and using medical technology, is linked to the Enlightenment in the late eighteenth century. An interesting phenomenon to notice is that the status of doctors in general became high in the social hierarchy from the time of the Enlightenment, because the development of science changed the image of the 'intelligentsia' and doctors although working in a practical field began to be recognised as part of this class, even though only a handful of doctors in theoretical fields had such a high standing in former ages. The doctor, on the whole, became able to earn prestige and economic power, and began to control the hospitals which were becoming reformed as institutions under professional authority. In relation to the improvement of the doctor's status in line with the development of scientific technologies, in the middle of the late eighteenth century, medical surgery in Britain developed remarkably. In the early nineteenth century, surgeons became able to have their own college (see Chapter 4 for fuller details). The doctors and modern medicine since the Enlightenment have been concerned with the improvement of practical and scientific aspects of medicine in terms of the treatment of the patient, which made their status higher, while disregarding theoretical fields such as the philosophical as well as the ethical aspects of medicine. Consequently, hospitals were increasingly becoming 'cure-centred', and so there arose the clear distinction between the hospice as one form of the medieval care-centred hospital, and the modern cure-centred hospital. It was also the time when many special hospitals such as cancer hospitals were established. Through the doctor's interest in the 'cure' of disease, 'death' tended to be understood merely as a defeat of medicine or science, which is unacceptable and disgraceful.

The Attitude to the Hospice in the Nineteenth Century

Although cancer hospitals in the nineteenth century tried to institute 'hospices' independent from any religious implication under the name of 'Friedenheims' which demonstrated a recognition of the needs of the dying, they came to nothing. This was because 'the demands for the support of clinical research into cancer were given more priority, in the hope that discovery of a cure would remove the need for such places as 'Friedenheims'' (Murphy, 1989, p.221). To accept the hospice seemed to mean to admit the defeat of medicine and science, so cancer hospitals, 'recognising that research would attract greater support than the care of the dying, shelved their Friedenheim plans and opened research laboratories'. Other cancer hospitals founded in various British cities tended to follow the pattern of paying attention to finding the medical cure for cancer. X rays were discovered at the end of 1895 and were first used in the treatment of cancer in 1896 (Murphy, 1989, pp.221-29). As hospices were replaced by hospitals, the holistic focus of the medieval hospice began to be neglected (Munley, 1983, p.29).

The Struggle in the Period of Modern Medicine

Herbert Snow, a consulting surgeon of the London Cancer Hospital, succeeded in using a mixture of opium and cocaine for cancer pain relief and published his research results in 1896 (Snow, 1896, p.718; cited by Murphy, 1989, p.227). Although this mixture became the basis of the Brompton cocktail, which would have an important role in the modern hospice care for the dying about seventy years later, no special notice was taken of this at the time (Murphy, 1989, pp.226-27).

In 1902, the Imperial Cancer Research Fund (ICRF) was established with a great expectation that 'cancer would be cured as a result of the work of scientists in its laboratories' (Murphy, 1989, p.227). During the Second World War, with the introduction of the medical treatment of cancer, aggressive treatments were reinforced even more by 'new antibiotics and synthetic hormones aimed at cure' (Infield, 1974; cited by Murphy, 1989, p.234). Consequently, by the 1960s, people were tending to die in hospital rather than in their homes (Murphy, 1989, p.234).

In the great progress of cancer treatment in the 1960s, patients and their families began to doubt whether aggressive treatment was really better than the disease itself. The question was raised about the worth of life prolongation if this was to mean continuous dramatic pain and suffering for a long time before death. Stoddard expresses his views of excessive life-prolongation at the university hospital in a dramatic way:

> ... The ICU is a supercomputer, a biochemical celebration, a sound-and-light show. It is also something like a launching pad. Disconnected from every familiar form of human contact and every ordinary support system, the patients lie one by one, espaliered, wired and turned like astronauts. (Stoddard, 1979, p.1; cited by Hill, 1989, p.4)

Against such inhuman treatment for the dying, the modern hospice movement started.

The Modern Hospice Movement

Hospice care survived through political as well as social changes by the effort of religious groups. During the seventeenth century in Britain, Sir Thomas Guy began a network of charitable hospitals, and Vincent de Paul (1581-1660) founded the hospice for galley slaves in France. Paul also founded an orphanage and established a Roman Catholic nursing order called 'the Sisters of Charity', dealing with nursing and teaching. By the eighteenth century the Sisters of Charity had founded hospices all over France, which revived the old philosophy of caring for the sick and dying with respect and compassion. Florence Nightingale was working with the Sisters of Charity in the nineteenth century. The actual idea of caring particularly for the dying in the hospice seemed to begin in the Dublin Hospice in the nineteenth century, where the old tradition of hospice care was transformed to a new understanding of the needs of the dying. In 1905 St Joseph's Hospice was established by the Sisters of Charity from Ireland in response to the intolerable conditions in London's East End, and the first patient was admitted in the same year (Manning, 1984, pp.40-42).

Without these Christian foundations which survived through the time of the Enlightenment and industrial revolution, the immediate development of the modern hospice movement from the 1960s might have been difficult. But on the other hand, the great hospice development since the 1960s until today is not imaginable either without the efforts of Cicely Saunders. Cicely Saunders was the first person who began to unite the old hospice concepts with methods of modern medical science, and took an important part in improving the methods of pain-control at St Joseph's. She opened St Christopher's hospice in London in 1968, which provides inpatient-care, home-care, and bereavement services, being partly financially supported by the National Health Service (Munley, 1983, p.29). In 1991, there were over 430 hospices in Britain, compared with less than fifteen in 1965 (James and Field, 1992, p.1363), and the concept of the hospice began to spread to the United States in the early 1970s (Munley, 1983, p.46).

Another important figure is Dr Kubler-Ross, who has been internationally known as one of pioneers in the research field of death, dying, and bereavement. Her famous book, 'On Death and Dying', was published in 1969, almost at the same time as the establishment of St Christopher's hospice in London by Cicely Saunders in 1968. Fulton describes the meaning of Kubler-Ross's work for the hospice movement:

We believe that it is correct to say that the initial responsibilities of American audiences to the hospice message of compassionate care and the relief of pain was conditioned in great part by the work of Dr Elisabeth Kubler-Ross and particularly by her book, *On Death and Dying*, which exposed a sensitive nerve in the health care delivery system of the United States ... This widely read book crystallized for the hospital nurse in particular the problems faced by those whose task was to deal with the private issues of death in a public setting. Her important and timely message to nurses and other care-givers across the country touched their hearts as it reached the public's ears and the effect was electrifying. (Fulton, 1981, p.10)

Not only in the United States as mentioned above but also in various different countries in the Western world, many founders of and researchers on the hospice have been deeply influenced by Kubler-Ross's work no matter whether they approve or disapprove of her theories of the care of the terminally ill and those in bereavement. It has become well-known that through her interviews with many dying patients, Kubler-Ross presented five stages in the dying process, which we will explain in the next chapter 'The Western Attitude to Death and Dying'. So we cannot ignore her existence in the development of the hospice in the Western world. Yet we do not intend to focus on her ideas in this chapter, despite the fact that they have become well known both by professionals or researchers in the field of death and palliative care and by lay people.

The main reason for this is that one of the most important purposes of this chapter is to discover the underlying religious ideas and symbolism found in the modern Western hospice philosophy but Kubler-Ross is not responsible for the hospice philosophy in this regard. She had already developed her research before the hospice arrived in the United States from Britain in 1970s, which means that her work is independent from the movement. Her theories have been of much practical use in the Western hospice, but what she was actually proposing was not 'hospice care'. She founded the centre for the terminally ill in California naming it 'Shanti Nilaya' (Sanskrit for 'Home of Peace'). Manning tends to identify this centre with the hospice in terms of its philosophy (Manning, 1984, p.57). But its intention was different even if it was doing the same at a practical level or had similar perspectives on death and dying, because the hospice has developed under such a deep Christian influence. In other words, the nature of care in 'Shanti Nilaya' cannot imply hidden religious symbolism as seen in the hospice movement which we will be exploring later in this chapter, even if it produces similar care for the dying as the hospice does. So Kubler-Ross's study has contributed to the hospice movement and she herself seems to encourage the hospice, but what she is doing cannot be called 'hospice care' because of its philosophical background. Our focus in this and later chapters is always on hospice care, so we cannot bring her study into the centre of our discussion, although we will refer it from time to time throughout the book.

Having looked at the history of the hospice movement from medieval to modern times in relation to the changes in the concept of the hospital, we come to understand that in the medieval age the idea of the hospice was not really distinguishable from the hospital. A clear distinction began to appear through the process of medicalization of the hospital from the time of the Black Death in the fourteenth century to the early nineteenth century. From the 1960s the modern hospice movement has been developed against the 'cure-centred' aggressive hospital treatment with its strong dependence upon scientific and technological equipment, which extends patients' lives and pain meaninglessly. The hospice movement has, however, disapproved of active euthanasia, and this attitude has brought about a paradox with the hospice's emphasis on the autonomy of the patient and pain-control, which we will discuss more in a later section. We now move to the next discussion on important issues related to the Western hospice movement, firstly the difficulty in the idea of the hospice as a philosophy of care, secondly the problems in the metaphorical relationship between 'pilgrims' and 'cancer patients', and finally the issue of voluntary euthanasia.

Is the Hospice a Philosophy of Care?   Four Criticisms

It has become understood that the hospice is not merely a building but a philosophy of care (Clark, 1993, p.169). (It needs to be clarified that the term 'philosophy' is not intended here to mean 'academic philosophy' but more a 'concept' or 'idea'.) We would like to discuss four main criticisms of the fact that the hospice has not yet become a real philosophy of care, which will help us to explore the nature of the modern hospice movement in the West:

A focus only on cancer patients;
Prejudice and discrimination against certain patients;
The emphasis on traditional forms of in-patient care;

The public support for a 'building' not a 'philosophy'.

As these issues, particularly the first three, are more closely related to practical aspects of hospice care, we will consider the more philosophical ones in a later section on the 'Pilgrim-Cancer Patient Metaphor'.

A Focus only on Cancer Patients

If the hospice is a philosophy of care, it must be applicable not only to cancer but to diseases of all kinds. Despite this, as Nicky James and David Field have pointed out, the hospice has been 'relatively specific with concentration on people dying of cancer', and 'for some people, hospices have become synonymous with 'dying of cancer'' (James and Field, 1992, p.1366). Why have cancer patients particularly attracted hospice care?

According to Seale's research 'Death from Cancer and Death from Other Causes' shows that the care of cancer patients is likely to be carried out over a short period but with a degree of intensity, and this suits the nature of hospice care. The hospice's emphasis on family involvement is also more relevant in the case of cancer, since families of cancer patients tend to be still alive. Because of the informal nature of cancer care, which is more likely to require psychological support than technical medical skills, the home care service provided by home care teams is also more appropriate for cancer than any other disease. Moreover, bereavement services supplied by many hospices are suitable for cancer, as relatives of the deceased are likely to be still alive (Seale, 1991a, pp.17-18).

Prejudice and Discrimination against Certain Patients

The hospice should, if it is a philosophy of care in general, not create a 'sacred area', where only a certain kind of patient enjoys the care; however, there has been criticism that hospices tend to exclude AIDS patients and also those from the black and ethnic minorities (Clark, 1993, p.172). Clark observes that 'too often hospices appear as white, middle class, Christian institutions serving a carefully selected group of patients' (1993, p.172). Carlisle has reported that doctors are sometimes deliberately making up evidence of cancer in AIDS patients so that they can gain support from charities (Carlisle, 1992, p.7).

The Emphasis on Traditional Forms of In-patient Care

According to the *Oxford Advanced Learner's Dictionary of Current English*, one of the definitions of the term 'philosophy' is 'a set of beliefs ... that is a guiding principle for behaviour' (p.928) and 'a building' is 'a structure with a roof and walls' (p.148). 'A set of beliefs' should exist without 'a building'; in other words, you can carry 'a philosophy' within yourself to wherever you want. On the other hand, you cannot usually carry 'a structure with a roof and walls' but need to bring yourself to where it is. It is of course possible to work for patients inside a building following the hospice philosophy, but it may not be called 'a philosophy' of care if what is meant by the hospice philosophy is not applicable outside the building.

According to Clark's survey of 43 new hospices in Britain, 79 per cent of them desired to establish some form of in-patient care, and only 16 per cent planned day-care only without any dependence on in-patient care though 90 per cent were planning for some day-care. While the interest in day-care is increasing enormously as this research shows, it does not decrease the aspiration for in-patient services. This shows the tendency of the hospice movement to relate to 'a building' rather than 'a philosophy' has not significantly changed since the middle of the 1980s (Clark, 1993, p.169).

The Public Support for a 'Philosophy of Care Only Inside Buildings' not a 'Philosophy of Care Everywhere'

There are currently over 400 hospice buildings in Britain, and they have been supported by the National Health Service (NHS) and charitable giving (Clark, 1993, p.170). The great support from charities means that the general public is aware of the need for hospice care, but whether the public supports the hospice philosophy on its own or the philosophy available only inside buildings is uncertain. This question arises when we consider the fact that the hospice philosophy is not really reflected in the public attitude to death or related issues. For example, British society is not yet open about emotional issues particularly those related to death such as bereavement, as Manning describes well:

> [O]ur society's difficulty with the expression of natural emotions and this is
> highlighted so clearly in the dilemma faced by a bereaved person ... She is
> permitted to cry and act 'irrationally' for only a very short time after the

funeral. After that any open display of expressive emotion is viewed with nervous embarrassment and interpreted as a morbid preoccupation rather than healthy release. The bereaved person is told to 'pull yourself together,' or 'to try to get back to normal' by well-meaning friends and relatives who will often not admit to themselves the embarrassment and fear they feel about such intense displays of emotion. (Manning, 1984, p.90)

If the huge number of hospice buildings implies that people encourage their society to pursue the hospice philosophy, this may have a strong influence on their attitude to death. The hospice has always tried to have an open attitude to death and dying, and the related emotional issues like bereavement. If the emotion of bereavement is still taboo in the society as described above, we suggest that there is a contradiction between the public's active support for the hospice movement and their attitude to bereavement. We may then need to regard the more than 400 hospices in Britain which have resulted from charitable giving as only establishing 'the buildings in which the hospice philosophy can be pursued' but not having changed the public attitude to death, dying, and bereavement or emotions through its philosophy.

This may be reflected also in the fact that incurable patients in hospitals are highly unlikely to know the prognosis of their disease, though they usually know its nature. While doctors and nurses in hospitals have become increasingly open about communicating with the terminally ill in terms of telling the name of the disease, partly through being influenced by the hospice movement, this does not often extend to telling the prognosis (Seale, 1991b, pp.943-952). It seems that doctors and nurses in hospitals are not yet open to the issue of death itself and not used to dealing with emotions experienced by patients and themselves in telling the prognosis. The hospice care philosophy has not yet extended far enough to influence the public and the hospital in respect of death and bereavement or other emotional issues, so we tend to see the great public support for the hospice movement as support for hospice care only inside the building or the institution, as it provides what people cannot gain in their society otherwise. We will explore this paradoxical situation more in the next section on 'the Pilgrim-Cancer Patient Metaphor'.

The Pilgrim-Cancer Patient Metaphor

Cicely Saunders, a leader of the modern hospice movement, chose the name 'hospice' when she established St Christopher's Hospice in London, where symptom control, psychological as well as spiritual support for cancer patients and their families, and also bereavement counselling were emphasized. As we explained in Section 1, however, the origin of the word 'hospice' simply meant 'a guest', 'host', or 'stranger' and did not have any implication of the dying or cancer patient. The use of the name 'hospice' for institutions caring for cancer patients might be considered as a conscious attempt to underline the link between medieval and modern hospices, as James and Field pointed out:

> The term 'hospice' was deliberately chosen and adopted by institutions caring for the terminally ill both to evoke the medieval way station for spiritual travellers and to differentiate them from ordinary hospitals (in Saunders, 1984). Thus the terminology of 'hospice' is itself an indication of the spiritual underpinning of the movement - an underpinning reinforced at some hospice conferences by prayers at the start of proceedings. Reports from overseas hospices also indirectly indicate the significance of organised religion, and Christianity in particular, in giving impetus to the hospices. (James and Field, 1992, p. 1366)

Although the expression 'deliberately' has a rather negative sense and may not be a relevant word to use in a factual enquiry about the hospice movement, we suggest that the above description might not be incorrect to the extent that there seems a tendency for modern hospices to connect the image of the medieval hospices with themselves. Considering the connection between the two, we might also see the image of medieval pilgrims replaced by that of cancer patients. Let us analyze in this section how strong the influence is of the metaphorical relationship between medieval and modern hospices on the one hand, and pilgrims and cancer patients on the other, on the philosophy of modern hospice care, and let us consider also the strength as well as the weakness of the metaphor in its application to terminal care. The analysis will highlight one of the most important problems of Western hospice care from a philosophical point of view.

The Image of Cancer

In the preceding section 'Is the hospice a philosophy of care?', we discussed why the modern hospice has been attracted particularly to cancer patients, but the reasons introduced were relatively practical ones. There would seem also to be some philosophical reasons to be considered as shown by the pilgrim-cancer patient metaphor, because the reason why cancer patients are associated with the modern hospice has to do with our attitude to cancer in relation to the Christian interpretation of pain. The Western image of cancer and Christian idea of pain, redemption, and salvation could create the pilgrim-cancer patient metaphor and are also vital in the modern hospice movement. Therefore we need to elucidate the image of cancer before going on to the argument about the strength and the weakness of the metaphor.

The Christian Interpretation of Illness Illness in general has had a strong link with the idea of sin in the West, and this seems to be related to the Christian religion. Kidel insists that 'our desire to be perfectly healthy implies an aspiration to divine status, a release from the bonds of mere humanity', and that 'there is still, in our times, an association between 'health' and 'virtue' on the one hand, 'illness' and 'sin' on the other' (Kidel, 1988, pp.6-7). To be healthy is the duty of Christians (Turner, 1987, p.23). The body, the flesh part of us which is regarded as something existing separately from our mind, is to be mastered; in other words, we humans are not allowed to be like animals acting according to their appetites, but must control them. To become ill means that we lose control over our bodily parts and become unable to do 'our duty' as a Christian, and this may be a sin. Pascal regarded his illness as a punishment and himself almost as a penitent who needed to repent his sins through the suffering produced by his illness as seen in his 'Prière pur le bon usage des maladies' (Prayer for Making Good Use of Illness) of 1654:

> Thou gavest me health to serve Thee, and I have used it only for worldly ends. Now Thou hast sent me illness in order to correct me. Do not permit me to use it to irritate Thee by my impatience. I have made bad use of my health, and Thou hast justly punished me for it; do not let me make bad use of Thy punishment. (Pascal, 1946, p.110; cited by Herzlich and Pierret, 1987, p.140)

During and after the eighteenth century, the time of the Enlightenment, as medical science developed and the church's power began to relax, the notion of sin and redemption was weakened. But the idea of sin and punishment in relation to illness is still often expressed in the same way, detached from religious meanings. In modern society, the origin of this attitude to illness may be forgotten but the notions remain.

The Understanding of Cancer - a Disease of Threefold Guilt (i) Patient's Guilt Any disease may carry the implication of sin and punishment, but in the case of cancer the idea is even stronger than in other diseases. There are a lot of anthropological as well as psychological reasons for this, but let us discuss just four main reasons.

The first is the dramatic pain of cancer over the long period of its terminal stage. Moreover, the patient often suffers not only from the disease itself but also from aggressive treatments, and both doctors and patients often express the thought that 'the treatment is worse than the disease' (Sontag, 1978, p.68). He or she might, for example, lose a part of the body such as a breast, leg, etc., and also lose his or her appetite after radiotherapy. In the hospice movement, the aspect of symptom control has been dramatically developed and all the aggressive treatments have been rejected, but some of the terminal pain is still thought of as uncontrollable, as we will describe later in the section on 'The hospice movement and voluntary euthanasia'. When we think of pain as an instrument of redemption, an uncontrollable pain must mean 'a lasting activity of redemption' until death. Cancer patients, who are 'called' to repent of their sin in this intolerable way, might be regarded as deadly sinners.

The second reason, which relates to the first is that cancer is often understood as 'a death penalty' since the disease is often incurable and one of the most common causes of death in the modern civilised Western world. Even if you try to 'make good use of God's punishment', suffering from the disease for your salvation, only death awaits you in the end. You have to suffer continuously for a long time but what you can gain is only death. Without a strong faith in going to heaven after the long term pain, you might find it difficult to feel the pain as an instrument for salvation. It seems, therefore, that to have cancer implies something more punitive than redemptive or salvational, because the patient sometimes suffers endlessly and only death can stop his physical pain.

Thirdly, cancer may be considered as a result of repression of negative emotions. There is a strong view of cancer as 'a disease of the failure of expressiveness' (Sontag, 1978, p.52) and repression of emotion (p.43). Also, 'certain psychologists and psychoanalysts believe that cancer has its origin in the individual history and the psychological characteristics of the subject' (Herzlich and Pierret, 1987, p.62). Reich even proposed a theory of cancer as an illness of repression of sexual energy (Reich, 1975; cited in Herzlich and Pierret, 1987, p.62). Moreover, Groddeck claims that the person himself creates his or her illness (Herzlich and Pierret, 1987, p.62). What is important here is not the question of whether or not the cause of cancer can be psychological stresses, but the fact that there is such a strong image of cancer as a result of repression of negative emotions. In this understanding of cancer, to prevent the disease, you should not repress stressful emotions in any circumstances of life, while emotional issues must be dealt with privately within you because of the Western difficulty in expressing emotions as we have seen in the quotation from Manning (1984, p.90; pp.14-15 above). It may be considered to be your fault when you get cancer 'as a consequence of repressing your emotions' which you have failed to control in a healthy way.

The fourth reason is the fact that cancer attacks people of different ages, sex, social class, and so on. Sontag explains that 'no one asks 'Why me?'of those who get cholera or typhus. But 'why me?' (meaning 'it's not fair') is the question of many who learn they have cancer' (Sontag, 1978, p.42). When you have cancer pain (punishment) despite having no particular sin in your present and past, you may begin to say 'Why me?' Just to be a good person or to live in a certain way seems to be no guarantee of safety from cancer, so cancer patients are those who are chosen 'by God'. Although the other diseases may also be regarded more or less as a punishment, the idea might be stronger in the case of cancer particularly for the four main reasons we have looked at.

The Understanding of Cancer - a Disease of Threefold Guilt (ii) Doctor's Guilt The social standing of Western doctors became increasingly high with the development of medical science, which increased man's knowledge of curing diseases as we will explore in Chapter 4. Since the Enlightenment, doctors have been thought of as leaders of science as well as healers, who could cure all diseases. But the existence of incurable cancer shows a limit to medical science and doctors as healers. Doctors cannot help admitting their defeat as scientists and curers when they have to face the reality that they are totally incapable in front of patients with incurable cancer. The defeat of science may mean that of doctors as well, because their high status has been attributed to the birth and progress of science. As scepticism grows about medical science, the status of doctors may become frail. While doctors may well desire to destroy scepticism, they can only give aggressive cure-centred treatments to the patients. Facing the patient dying of cancer with a lot of pain from the disease and the treatments, the doctor feels guilty about his inability to help him or her out of pain and death.

The Understanding of Cancer - a Disease of Threefold Guilt (iii) Family's Guilt The patient's family may also feel guilty about watching their loved one suffering from the disease and painful treatments. In cure-centred modern hospitals, the family are not allowed to take part in the treatment of the patient, partly because the treatment tends to be professional as it requires special knowledge and skill. It must be painful to the family just to look at their loved one in pain without being able to release him or her from agony, and leaving him or her to the medical staff.

It might be possible to call cancer 'a disease of threefold guilt'. Cancer patients are those who have failed to control their emotions properly, so are not to be respected, while being given up on by their doctors and families. We may call a cancer patient a 'deserted, disrespected, and punished sinner'. As to 'desertion', however, it does not mean that doctors and families really want to 'desert' the patient but are almost forced to give up their embrace in the traditional process of hospitalization, and this might be why it was necessary to create another environment involving the idea of care, such as the hospice for cancer patients.

A Comparison between Medieval Pilgrims and Modern Cancer Patients

The aim here is to understand the difference and similarity between medieval pilgrims and cancer patients, as it will help us later to see how the pilgrim-cancer patient metaphor works in the hospice movement and to explore problems which tend to arise when the pilgrim's image is metaphorically linked with cancer patients. The comparison will be made in the following aspects:

> the idea of sin and pain;
> closeness to death;
> the matter of choice;
> the idea of the 'stranger';
> care-only and care-centred.

The Idea of Sin and Pain (i) 'Pilgrimage' as a Penance Pilgrimage was often forced upon people as a penance or even as civil and criminal law penalties in the ninth century during the reigns of Popes Nicholas I (858-

67) and Stephen V (885-91), because it involved many difficulties in travelling abroad. Pilgrimages were made also for curing diseases, and this could not be totally separated from the idea of 'penance', since in Christianity the idea of sin is often connected with that of pain and disease, as already stated (Kendall, 1970, pp.17-19).

When we believe that our spiritual and physical pains are caused by our sin, the forgiveness of the sin may result in the relief of the pain. Jesus linked the notion of forgiving people and their sins with that of healing them, where the idea of healing as wholeness brings out the two aspects as combined. So it seems that the idea of seeking for forgiveness of sins and for the cure of diseases at the end of their journey became merged within the purpose of the pilgrimage. Until reaching the shrine and obtaining forgiveness of sins, pilgrims had not yet been forgiven; in other words, they were still 'sinners' unless they had atoned for their sins by completing their journey as a penance.

The Idea of Sin and Pain (ii) The Christian Mission and 'Jesus' within Pilgrims We need to consider now why medieval hospices treated those who were 'not yet redeemed sinners' warmly and kindly as if they had been 'Jesus'. Three reasons are considered there. Firstly, medieval hospices built by Christian orders had a mission to help 'sinners (pilgrims)' to complete their journey so that their soul would be saved by the forgiveness of sins and their disease would be cured at the end of their journey. Secondly, the hospices tried to find the image of Jesus, who carries a cross on his shoulder, within all pilgrims continuing their journey with difficulties and the aspiration for their sins to be forgiven and their diseases cured. In fact Jesus said in the New Testament, 'I was a stranger and ye took me in' (Matthew 25: 35). This teaches that Jesus exists in every stranger, and that helping a stranger in pain is the same as helping Jesus. Thirdly, they are 'not yet redeemed sinners' but penitents, and penitents are welcomed by God even more than good people in the Christian idea, as the parable of 'the lost sheep' of the New Testament shows (Matthew 18: 10-14).

The Idea of Sin and Pain (iii) Cancer Patients as Sinners Cancer patients could be also, to some extent, regarded as 'sinners' in the modern age, but modern hospices treat them as 'guests' to be respected. The dying process of cancer patients may be thought as the time for preparation for death. In the Christian tradition people need to atone for sin before death, otherwise they are supposed to go to hell or purgatory. Modern hospices try to help cancer patients to complete 'a pilgrimage to death' satisfactorily. One of the most important aspects of hospice care is physical pain relief, and when the patient's physical pain is appropriately controlled he or she can think about their life and death; what they regret or feel guilty about; what they want to achieve in the rest of their life; etc. Such reflection is in tune with Kubler-Ross's idea of psychological pain relief through completing 'unfinished business', in which she encourages patients to express the unexpressed emotions of anger, loss, etc (Manning, 1984, p.56).

Although in the modern hospice all this reflection and contemplation may no longer be done particularly for the redemption of sins or salvation after death, nor in a strong awareness of Christian faith, at least it gives great peace to patients if done with the psychological support of their family and caring staff. The process of reflecting on one's past life is often painful psychologically and spiritually, since patients often have to face the harsh reality in their life of no significant achievement, unsuccessful human relationships, and so on. Hospice care may help them to reach a peaceful state of mind after some painful reflection on their previous life and on their death by dealing with or accepting their anger and fear with the destiny of death. Patients may be able to find 'a jewel' even from a miserable life and to feel their life to have been meaningful and graceful. To have a peaceful state of mind may mean that patients forgive themselves and others (including God) accepting all the events (including their incurable disease) in the past and present life totally. The psychological process before this state tends to remind us of the journey of medieval pilgrims to the shrine for the sake of the forgiveness of sins. Whether the forgiveness is given by God or the individuals themselves, medieval pilgrims and modern 'cancer pilgrims' are linked together in terms of awareness of 'being forgiven' after a long and difficult journey in mind and body. One of the crucial purposes of hospice care in both medieval and modern times seems, therefore, to be to help 'pilgrims' to obtain 'the forgiveness of sins' in the way which we have described, though there is no guarantee that this purpose is achieved particularly in the case of the modern hospice.

Closeness to Death Medieval pilgrims had to carry on their travel whilst in great danger of picking up plague, and meeting thieves and robbers. In other words, their travel was always close to death (Kendall, 1970, pp.52-5). The following verse from a pilgrim hymn expresses this:

You who are going to Santiago,
I humbly beg you
Make no haste:
Go your way gently.
Alas! how the poor sick folk
Are in great discomfort!
For many men and women
By the wayside are dead.
(translated in Kendall, 1970, p.55; from King, 1920)

Modern cancer patients are of course close to death, since their admission for hospice care means that their death in the near future is almost definite. However, there is a difference between medieval pilgrims and modern cancer patients in the extent of the predictability of death. The former still had some hope of surviving until reaching the shrine although death must indeed have been a day-to day event as the poem shows, but the latter have a certainty of death, as it is more possible to predict that one's cancer is incurable, and how long the rest of life will last than with most other diseases. The purpose of the medieval pilgrimage and the 'pilgrimage' of a cancer patient might have some similarity as we discussed earlier, but they differ in the actual destination of the 'journey' since the destination of medieval pilgrims was a shrine while that of cancer patients is an unavoidable death. So the closeness of death to the pilgrims was whilst they were on their way to the destination and there was always some hope of survival, but to cancer patients, it was at the destination and there is almost no hope of surviving. Although both medieval pilgrims and cancer patients are close to death, the nature of anxiety, fear, and loneliness connected to their 'journey' might be different in relation to the predictability and the time of death, as seen in the above.

The Matter of Choice It is not easy to discern whether or not a decision about going on a pilgrimage by medieval pilgrims was made only by their free will. As already mentioned, one of the biggest reasons for the medieval pilgrimage was to obtain the forgiveness of sins, and taking the journey was sometimes required even as a penance or penalty. If you had been a Christian at that time, you would have made your pilgrimage for your salvation - 'We are sinners, so need to be forgiven by God'. Unless you made a pilgrimage, you might not be saved. In a way, therefore, medieval pilgrims did not have choice, particularly if the pilgrimage had been made as a penance or penalty. It appears then to have been compulsory in those days, when the Christian religion had a strong political power over people's daily life. However, on the other hand, when we understand that this apparently compulsory pilgrimage was a vocation for Christians of those days, the question of choosing to become a pilgrim would be far more complicated, because the concept of 'must', 'desire', and 'want' could not be perfectly distinguished, as shown below:

a. I am a sinner, so *must* make my pilgrimage for my salvation.

b. Why must you?

a. Because God wants me to do so, and I *must* follow His will.

b. You can ignore the will of God if you wish.

a. Yes, I can, but I won't because I *want* to follow His will by my free will.

b. Why do you want to follow His will?

a. Because I *want* salvation, but I am a sinner, so must make my pilgrimage.

In the psychological mechanism of vocation, as shown, we can understand the reason of pilgrimage neither by 'must' nor by 'want' alone, since the will of God and that of a human interact with each other. When you are 'called' to be a pilgrim by the will of God, you should feel you want to be so. In regard to cancer patients, we looked at cancer whose cause has sometimes been regarded as the patient's own fault through the repression of emotion, a failure to control emotion, bad deeds in the past, etc. It might be difficult, however, to call it a vocation, since there seems no room for the 'wants' of the individual; that is to say, no one wants to get cancer. Even in the case of a lung cancer patient who is a heavy smoker, we cannot say that he wanted to get cancer, though we may be able to say that he chose to be a heavy smoker despite knowing there was a great risk of getting lung cancer due to his smoking. The word 'vocation' should imply the concept of 'want' though it cannot be perfectly distinguished from 'must', and therefore pilgrims still have room to choose about their journey (except for the case in which pilgrimages were enforced as a criminal penalty by the law). Here there might be a crucial distinction between pilgrims and cancer patients with regard to the possibility of their decision making for their 'pilgrimage'. Medieval hospices cared for pilgrims who were often 'called' to the journey and said 'yes' to their destiny whether it was harsh or fatal, but modern hospices have to care for those who are often angry with their destiny of death from cancer or the betrayal of their bodies (Munley, 1983, p.97, pp.162-164, p.199).

The Idea of the 'Stranger' Christianity has emphasized the idea that we find Jesus within each person whether he or she is a stranger or even an enemy. As shown in an earlier section, the Latin 'hospes' which is the origin of the English word 'hospice' began to take on the meaning of 'stranger' under the Christian influence in the medieval age. Medieval hospices were shelters for strangers such as pilgrims who had no help on the road away from their family. So they needed to be cared for by kind strangers at a hospice. The pilgrim's status was as an 'outsider' or 'stranger' there, and this suited the idea of medieval hospice care, which is deeply related to Christian altruism even toward 'strangers'.

On the other hand, in the modern period, cancer patients often have their relatives around them at the hospice. The hospice was a place for strangers who were cared for by strangers, but in the modern hospice, cancer patients are cared for not only by strangers but also by their family. So the status of cancer patients could not be as strangers on the road who have no acquaintances around them. The question here is whether the name 'hospice' is appropriate for a shelter for cancer patients who are with their family. In addition, we may need to be concerned about the risk that cancer patients are forced to be 'strangers' within the society, when they are provided with hospice care and become 'pilgrims'. We will consider this more later on.

Care-Only and Care-Centred Both medieval and modern hospices did/do emphasize 'care', but the situation in which the care was/is stressed is different. In medieval hospices, pilgrims were welcomed and given hospitality with no medical treatment being given to the inmates, but this does not mean that the medieval hospice respected 'care' in the way which modern hospices do. In the medieval hospices, they did not give any 'cure' not because of their philosophy but because of the undeveloped state of medicine in those days; in other words, they had *no choice* between whether they wanted to provide surgical operations etc. to cure patients' diseases or just hospitality. On the other hand, modern hospices respect a care-centred treatment for the dying, despite today's advanced medical technology applicable to 'cure-centred treatment' which can prolong the patient's life. Therefore, it is possible to give aggressive treatments, but hospices willingly *choose* care-centred medicine by definition.

The Strength of the Metaphor

If the term 'hospice' was intentionally chosen for the name of institutions caring for cancer patients, we suspect that the aim was to connect the image of the medieval hospices and pilgrims with that of modern hospices and cancer patients, whether consciously or unconsciously. In this part of Section 3, let us try to explore what sort of benefit cancer patients, their families, and carers can gain when the metaphor is involved in the philosophy of the modern hospice movement.

Purification of the Threefold Guilt The modern hospice movement has changed the image of cancer patients from 'deserted, disrespected, and punished sinners' into 'innocent pilgrims'. Why are pilgrims innocent? They may be also called 'sinners', since they went on a pilgrimage for the forgiveness of sin. We could say, however, that they are penitents, who are even more welcomed by God than good people are, as the parable of 'the lost sheep' (Matthew 18: 12-14) or 'the prodigal son' (Luke 15: 10-32) in the New Testament shows. When you become a penitent, you become more valuable than just being a sinner. The cancer patient becomes a penitent who travels shouldering his or her 'own cross', and in whom Jesus is, once the person is accepted to receive hospice care. As mentioned already, there is a tie between the forgiveness of sin for medieval pilgrims and gaining a peaceful state of mind in cancer patients after painful reflection and contemplation of their lives. In this context, it is understandable that modern hospices think that emotional support is one of the most important aspects of hospice care.

 With regard to doctors, they also do not have to feel guilty about their defeat as scientists or their inability to help cancer patients escape from pain and death, because of the redefinition of their role in terminal care. Doctors can find a more care-centred way of helping patients by developing pain-control medicine, communication skills for psychological care of the dying, etc. (Particularly concerning pain-control medicine, doctors can keep their status as a professional person since the pain-control must be done carefully and needs a special knowledge of drugs.) Furthermore, the family's feeling of guilt is reduced, because they can take a big part in caring for the patient in hospice care, which emphasizes informal care so the family can have a role in the treatment of the patient:

> Family members typically said that they fulfilled many tasks for their relatives both in the in-patient hospice and at home - from direct physical

care (such as feeding, turning, bathing, personal grooming) to providing small pleasures and diversions. The impact that direct participation may have on 'feeling positive about self' later is suggested by Mrs. Larson (a wife of a patient). (Munley, 1983, p.189)

The family no longer have just to stand beside the patient suffering from pain, leaving everything to medical staff, but can re-establish a family tie with the patient through this opportunity by sharing feelings with him or her and making him or her comfortable.

Modification of the Image of Death and Cancer for Carers When the expression 'the dying process' is replaced by 'pilgrimage' or 'journey'. and 'cancer patient' by 'pilgrim', the image of death and cancer may be modified. Cicely Saunders indeed stressed 'hospitality' for the patients. Suppose you are a doctor or a nurse or perhaps a voluntary worker for cancer patients, it might be psychologically easier for you if you feel the patients are travellers or pilgrims on the road and that your role is to give them 'hospitality' so they can end their journey peacefully. It must be psychologically difficult, however, if you feel them to be those dying of a disease of guilt full of pain. You might be able to identify yourself with the role as 'host' expected to give hospitality to 'pilgrims', rather than with the doctor or the nurse treating 'dying patients with an awful disease like a cancer'. Here the notions of 'death' and 'cancer' become rather indirect, and that will help carers dealing with cancer patients.

Previously, in the section on 'Is the Hospice a Philosophy?', we tried to understand why cancer patients attract hospice care, giving some relatively practical reasons, but now it seems possible to consider a theoretical reason in relation to the metaphorical relationship between medieval pilgrims and cancer patients; in other words, cancer is a disease which could be more easily connected metaphorically with 'pilgrims' than other diseases. Firstly, this is because cancer has been considered to be 'a disease of guilt'. Guilt and sin have been one of the most important subjects in Christianity, whose philosophy has always coexisted with hospice care, not only in medieval but also in modern times, as Saunders observed of St Christopher's:

We are not all Christians, by any means, but our work is done in obedience to the Christian imperative. For me personally, it could not be done otherwise. (Saunders, quoted by James and Field, 1992, p.1366 from Stoddard, 1979, p.74)

As far as the hospice philosophy is based upon Christian ideas, cancer will be an attractive disease for the modern hospice, because the disease seems to have a strong connection with the idea of sin and pain. Secondly, cancer patients do not usually die immediately, and the period of time before death could be analogically overlapped with the idea of 'a journey' made by medieval pilgrims.

Furthermore, the pilgrim-cancer patient metaphor makes 'death' itself valuable and meaningful because the destination of 'cancer pilgrims' is the same as that of Christ, that is, DEATH. What was waiting for Jesus after a long painful journey was death on the Cross, and the destination of 'cancer pilgrims' is also death. In this sense, cancer patients can be identified with Jesus on the way to his Cross even more than medieval pilgrims could be because, as we have explored already, medieval pilgrims' destinations were shrines, though the closeness and the danger of death were always existent on their journey. As Christ's death may make his painful journey have a profound meaning, the destination of 'death' of cancer patients may also do the same for their 'pilgrimages', and this identification may contribute to redefining the meaning of death and the status of cancer patients from a negative to a positive one.

The Weakness of the Metaphor

We have reached the most important part of this chapter now. We have seen that modern hospices seem to attempt to link the image of cancer patients with that of pilgrims. One result of such linking would be the new status of cancer patients raised to that of 'a penitent' who should be respected and valued in Christian teaching. Another is the reduction of the feeling of guilt on the part of the patients, families, and doctors. However, when pilgrims and cancer patients are forced to be metaphorically connected despite the difficulty in creating the metaphor, which we have shown earlier in our comparison between the two, some problems may appear. The problems are considered in relation to the following:

Producing a certain ideal way of death and dying;

The paradoxical relationship between hospice care and the public attitude to death.

Producing a Certain Ideal Way of Death and Dying (i) In Relation to 'Care-Only' and 'Care-Centred' Remembering the fifth aspect 'care-only and care-centred' which we discussed earlier, we need to look at the fact that the 'care' or 'hospitality' of medieval hospices and that of modern hospices is different and this may push cancer patients towards a certain way of death.   Modern hospices intentionally choose the care-centred approach despite the fact that the cure-centred way would be possible if they wished to follow it.   In the action of choosing something, a certain sense of value or a philosophy (which makes one choose something) is involved, and therefore it must be distinguished from the action of doing something because there is nothing otherwise.

Imagine I choose to go to London from Wales on foot not using any vehicle, because I think it good for my health.   There may also have been some people once upon a time who walked to London since it was the only way.   If I try to identify myself with these people through the meaning of the action 'go to London on foot', that may imply that I walk to London in this modern period as if it *were* the sole way.   My action of choosing the way of getting to London on foot can be hidden in the identification.   Likewise, modern hospices have *chosen* the care-centred treatment of the patients, with their ideals and values, but they could hide the action of 'choosing,' and make it appear as if their way were the only one.   In other words, the metaphor encourages us to feel that there is no choice but the hospice care ideal for the dying.   Therefore, the modern hospice creates the hospice way of death and dying, to the attitude to pain and suffering, emotions, euthanasia, etc.

When the different circumstances between the 'care-only' environment of the medieval hospice and the 'care-centred' policy of the modern hospice are ignored, the modern hospice way of death and dying and treating patients may appear to have an absolute value.   When the hospice care philosophy is given an absolute value by such a confusion between the idea of 'care-centred' and 'care-only', there is a risk that the hospice tries to create the notion of 'a good death' rather than just making the dying process more comfortable as well as peaceful.

Moreover, looking at the fact that hospice care may begin to be represented as more a specialized form of caring which may appear as another medical speciality called 'palliative care', we need to be worried about the danger that this notion of specialty (which might create a more institutionalised structure as in hospitals, where there is a strong hierarchy of carers and also the paternalism of doctors) might be justified by the metaphorical confusion between 'care-centred' and 'care-only'.   In other words, the hospices may keep giving an impression to the public that their way is the only way for the care of the dying even in the future when they may no longer be care-centred.

Producing a Certain Ideal Way of Death and Dying (ii) In Relation to the Matter of Choice   If medieval pilgrimages were a sort of vocation as a result of the interaction between God's will and the person's inclination, there seems to be room for the 'wants' of the individual, but the case of cancer patients does not leave such room.   Again, the metaphor might impose values in regard to the attitude to disease and death.   Why should cancer patients think of cancer as an 'instrument of salvation' or something similar which involves such hidden symbolism?   Why do they need 'the forgiveness of sin' or something similar?   They might have no idea of being 'punished' by getting such a disease as cancer.   Although cancer patients may rise up to the status of 'pilgrims', they are still 'penitents', who are asked to repent of their sins, despite the fact that they were never willing to be 'cancer pilgrims'.   Hospice care may not easily become independent from these Christian notions of pain and death, as long as the term 'hospice', which has such a strong Christian connotation included in the metaphor, is used.   This may, again, create a certain ideal way (perhaps the Christian way) of death and dying as caring staff may expect (even unconsciously) patients to achieve a certain sort (the Christian sort) of spiritual development.

The Paradoxical Relationship between Hospice Care and the Public Attitude to Death   We have come to understand the hospice movement as a strong reaction against the hospitalization of death, which treats only the physical side of patients but not the mental or psychological side; and provides unnaturally excessive life-prolongation through aggressive treatments.   On the other hand, there is a paradoxical relationship between hospice care and the public in terms of the attitude to death and dying, as the hospice movement might reinforce existing attitudes outside hospice care.   Let us draw out the following comparison so that the situation can be understood more clearly:

A. Outside hospice care

cancer patients as punished, deserted, and disrespected sinners

not respected not cared for, but avoided

the topic of death is taboo

death is defeat and dread

emotional issues are taboo

no psychological involvement with cancer patients

aggressive treatments in hospital

threefold guilt

B. Inside hospice care

cancer patients as pilgrims or penitents

respected, cared for, given 'hospitality'

the topic of death is not taboo

death has a profound value because of 'the cross' and 'pilgrimage'

emotional issues are not taboo

psychological involvement with cancer patients

no aggressive treatment

purification of threefold guilt

The expression 'hospice care' does not necessarily imply a building structure but whichever place hospice care occurs in: in hospice buildings, hospitals, homes, and so on. 'A. Outside hospice care' is therefore whichever place is not part of hospice care. We may spell out a logical explanation of the paradoxical relationship:

* there might not be the condition in **B** without the condition in **A**, against which **B** tries to react;

* in other words, the existence of condition **B**, in which cancer patients become 'pilgrims', is a kind of evidence of the existence of condition **A**;

* the pilgrim-cancer patient metaphor created in condition **B** is a kind of evidence of the condition **A**;

* because of the condition **A**, therefore, cancer patients have to become pilgrims;

* in the end, the pilgrim-cancer patient metaphor reinforces condition **A**.

In so far as the metaphor holds, cancer patients may remain 'pilgrims' who are strangers outside hospice care, because they are the objects of interest only to hospice care. We already suggested in the section 'Is the

Hospice a Philosophy of Care ?' that hospice care has not yet become 'a philosophy of care'.   Particularly, taking 'The public support for 'buildings' not 'philosophy of care'' into consideration, we suggested that the public or the world outside hospice care tends to support hospice buildings to send cancer patients on their 'pilgrimage' as 'travellers'.

There is a circle here.

1. Within condition **A**, people do not psychologically or physically get involved with cancer patients, but support (contribute money to) hospice care for the sake of the patients or for their own future when they or their family may get cancer - buying 'an indulgence'.

2. Because of 1, one becomes 'a pilgrim' when he or she gets cancer, and the number of pilgrims is increased.

3. However, situation 2 is a sort of reflection on condition **A**, which cannot itself resolve the problem.

4. Therefore, some problems remain to be solved outside hospice care (**A**).

5. Going back to 1, within condition **A**, people do not get involved with cancer patients, but support (contribute money to) hospice care for the sake of the patients or for their own future when they or their family may get cancer - buying 'an indulgence'.

6. Because of 1/5 ... .

The circle considered in this paradoxical relationship between hospice care and the world outside of hospice care could be compared to 'a greenhouse' and 'wasteland'. Because there is wasteland (outside hospice care) where you can grow nothing, you build a special greenhouse (hospice buildings or hospice care groups) and get strawberries (hospice care) from there. Many people living in the wasteland visit your greenhouse to get some fresh strawberries (in-patient hospice care) or, alternatively, you might go and visit the wasteland to distribute your strawberries to them (day care or home care organized by the hospice). But people may never try to cultivate the wasteland to grow strawberries because of their dependency upon your greenhouse (no significant change or openness in the public attitude to death, dying, and cancer). Or people may try to build many greenhouses like yours in the wasteland (the public interest in building more hospice buildings). The 'greenhouse' here is analogous with hospice care and strawberries are the hospice ideal of care as shown in condition **B**. The wasteland is the world outside of hospice care in condition **A**.

When we think of the huge number of hospice buildings or hospice care groups existing in Britain, it seems that a lot of 'greenhouses' have been built in the wasteland. We should acknowledge, however, that the 'greenhouse' is something special which is separated from the outside world. It is a place you do not want to visit until your 'May' (the time for your and your loved ones' death and your bereavement) comes and you need to eat some strawberries from there (receiving hospice care). In the greenhouse, you can grow strawberries (hospice care) even in 'December' (the time for others' death and bereavement) but outside you can never do so. When your neighbour next door says that he or she wants to eat strawberries (hospice ideal of care) because his or her 'May' has come, you might just say, 'Please go to the nearest greenhouse so you can eat strawberries', but you might never go together with your neighbour to the greenhouse (the public's closed attitude to death), because you think that *now* is not 'your May'. You know where to go *in your own May* when you desire to eat strawberries, but until then you shut yourself out from the house while maintaining it for your 'May' to come. Strawberries here mean the hospice way of caring for the dying, and 'May' means the time of your own dying or those close to you and also the time of your bereavement. 'December' is the time of others' dying and bereavement.

So the people (dying cancer patients) who go to 'greenhouses' (hospice care) are 'pilgrims', or 'strangers' in the modern age, whom you do not know how to deal with or are scared to get involved with. The home care service is increasingly developing in the hospice movement (Taylor, 1983, p.9; cited by Clark, 1991, p.997), and home carers ('gardeners') bring strawberries (the hospice-type care) from the greenhouse (the hospice institution) even if you do not go yourself to the greenhouse. No one would, however, need to get 'strawberries' from them until their 'May' (the time for death and bereavement of himself and his loved ones), but only those 'in their own May' need the 'gardeners' visit'. People in their own May tend to be isolated in the wasteland (the society outside hospice care), because society, as we have explored in A above, does not want to have any involvement with them. 'Gardeners' (carers from the hospice) are like the Good Samaritan (Luke 10: 25-37) who cares for 'strangers' (dying cancer patients in the society outside the hospice) on the road who have no help otherwise. Here, the pilgrim-cancer patient metaphor holds.

There is a movement now through which hospital care is becoming closer to hospice-type care (Seale, 1989, pp.551-59) without using the term 'hospice' but using the term 'palliative care' instead. However, methods of palliative care have been moved from hospices into general hospitals (Clark, 1993, p.176), so those dealing with palliative care in hospitals may come from the hospice organization or often have a background of working in hospices; in other words, palliative care in hospitals is still very much dependent upon hospices. Therefore, it seems that hospital palliative care could not be easily detached from the 'pilgrim-cancer patient metaphor'. It does not make any difference whether 'the greenhouse' is brought into hospitals or hospice buildings or homes, because the greenhouse is a place providing strawberries for certain people in their own May, and is avoided by others who have not yet reached their own May. Moreover, there might be a difficulty in bringing the hospice philosophy to hospitals, because the hospice was originally developed as a strong reaction against the way of treating the dying in hospital.

It is dangerous to say that the pilgrim-cancer patient metaphor is always significant in all Western hospices, and we have no intention of giving the reader the impression that modern Western hospices are merely part of a Christian movement, where no secularization is allowed. On the other hand, the value involved in the metaphor can remain even unconsciously in the secularized hospices, as we, for example, can use this metaphor in relation to the modern attitude to death and dying, in which the dying and the bereaved become 'strangers' within society.

The Hospice Movement and Voluntary Euthanasia

> [A]ll those who work with dying people are anxious that what is known already should become so good that no one need ever ask for voluntary euthanasia. (Saunders, 1972; cited by Glover, 1990, p.182)

> [N]o one should reach that desperate place where he could only ask for his life to be ended. (Saunders, 1977, p.8)

We tend to think that the above descriptions do not refer to 'voluntary passive euthanasia', remembering that one of Saunder's priorities for the hospice is 'relief of pain' which may be done for the patient even if it shortens his life. 'Ask for his life to be ended' is likely to imply that the person is asking for some active method to end his life, and this is different from asking for his life not to be prolonged by any active method or for pain-relief by frequent doses of a pain killer like morphine or the Brompton-cocktail which might shorten his or her life. So conceptually what Saunders means by voluntary euthanasia should not include passive euthanasia, though she suggests that the term 'passive euthanasia' is confusing and had better not be used (Saunders, 1980, pp.52-3). In this section, let us elucidate a conflict between the hospice and the idea of voluntary 'active' euthanasia rather than passive euthanasia.

The Problem Related to Legislation for Voluntary Euthanasia

The first Voluntary Euthanasia Society in the World was founded in 1935 by a number of distinguished doctors and laymen including the royal surgeon, Lord Moynihan. It was established for the purpose of promoting a Voluntary Euthanasia Legislation Bill proposed by Dr C. K. Millard from the Society of Medical Officers of Health in 1931. In the proposed Voluntary Euthanasia Act of 1969, individuals would have been allowed to sign a declaration form in advance, similar to that of a 'Living Will' (Wilson, 1975, pp.31-41). While 'Living Wills' have not yet been legally endorsed by statute in Britain, the British Medical Association has made a statement, urging doctors to respect such declaration forms when they have been completed (The Terrence Higgins Trust, 1992).

The British government tends to regard the hospice movement as an answer to the question of legislation for some form of active euthanasia. The following is from 'Salute to the Hospice Movement' signed by 181 members of Parliament:

> [T]his house salutes the success of all those involved in the hospice movement and in palliative care; congratulates those who care for the terminally ill and the dying on the great progress which has been achieved in the development of palliative care medicine in the United Kingdom; noted with profound concern the fact that in the Netherlands euthanasia now accounts for 3700 deaths each year of which more than 1000 are as a result of involuntary euthanasia; and registers its opposition to the decriminalisation of euthanasia in this country. ('Salute to the Hospice Movement', 1992, p.1571, cited by Clark, 1993, p.120).

The statement implies that the British government is likely to have a negative attitude to the legalization of euthanasia, with its concern for cases like those in the Netherlands, in which involuntary euthanasia has been shown to be taking place. In 1988, the British Medical Association also said, in its Report on Euthanasia: 'We feel that there is almost never a point at which an active intervention causing death is preferable to a natural death'. The American Medical Association declares: 'The intentional termination of the life of one human being by another - mercy killing - is contrary to that for which the medical profession stands and is contrary to the policy of the A.M.A.' (Beloff, 1993, p.4). The position in regard to active euthanasia seems to vary from one voluntary euthanasia society to another, but we would like to quote a description by Dr John Beloff, an ex-chairman and the present honorary secretary of the Voluntary Euthanasia Society of Scotland:

> Our movement may be said to have two primary objectives, the one positive, the other negative. The negative objective is to ensure that medical intervention will not be forcibly applied to keep people alive who want to be allowed to die in peace. The positive objective is to change the law so that a doctor may be allowed to respond to a patient's appeal to expedite his or her demise. (Beloff, 1993a, p.4)

The former, says Beloff, has been almost achieved by the Living Will, but the situation is difficult when we come to the positive objective, which seems to imply active euthanasia, as rejected by the BMA and AMA. But the Scottish Society still insists:

> [T]he hospice cannot possibly provide the answer to the demand to be allowed to die with dignity. As Ludovic Kennedy recently pointed out, there are only about 2000 hospice beds in this country whereas there are something like 150,000 deaths per year from cancer alone. Although our society has no party line and opinions may differ among our members, most of us, especially those on the Executive Committee, are in favour of changing the law so that doctors would be permitted to help patients to die if that was their expressed wish. (Beloff, 1993b)

The Scottish Society insists on the right to active euthanasia, which is against the policy of the hospice. But there are some societies with different attitudes to the issue. For example, in the Voluntary Euthanasia Society of West Australia, a member can choose the active or the passive route as he or she likes (Oki, 1991, p.286).

Cicely Saunders is strongly against legislation for voluntary euthanasia:

> I believe there is no way in which the few who would wish for euthanasia
> or instruction on how to kill themselves can be offered a 'quick way out'
> without society bringing pressures, conscious and unconscious, upon the
> many who are vulnerable ... To suggest that such an act should be legalised
> is to offer a negative and dangerous answer to problems which should be
> solved by better means. (Saunders, 1980, pp.52-3)

The Hospice and a Christian Perspective on Death and Pain

Through our discussion in an earlier section we saw that the modern
hospice has kept a Christian attitude to pain and suffering, and that its
attitude to the patient is also based upon Christian ideas. So we cannot
ignore Christian ethics when we consider the hospice's position to
voluntary active euthanasia. According to 'Directive 21' of the Ethical
and Religious Directives for Catholic Hospitals, all forms of Euthanasia
(mercy killing) are denied from the perspectives of the value of suffering
and the inviolability of human life (Wilson, 1975, p.82).

The Inviolability of Human Life This idea can be found in the expression
'The innocent and righteous slay thou not' (Exodus 23: 7). In the
Christian tradition, we have to apply this rule not only to others but
ourselves, so suicide is understood to be a deadly sin. Thomas Aquinas
understood suicide as the destruction of man's natural inclination to live
for the perfection of his being (Wilson, 1975, pp.82-83).

The Value of Suffering Sullivan argues against euthanasia on the basis of
the value of suffering. He claims that man's perfection is impossible
without suffering given by God according to each man's need. He insists
that God gives humans pain so that they can atone for their sins and be
closer to perfection through their sufferings, and that 'suffering is almost
the greatest gift of God's love' (Sullivan, 1950, p.57; cited by Wilson,
1975, p.83).

Both the perspectives contain the view that our life and death
including pain and suffering are at God's hand in the end, and this
corresponds well to the hospice attitude to voluntary active euthanasia.
The hospice also leaves the matter of death, life, and pain, to the hand of
God in the end. The hospice makes every effort to release the patient
from pain in their terminal stage, but there may be a sort of pain which

is not controllable. Ventafridda reports that it is not always possible to help the patient to die peacefully even in the hospice because 52.5 percent of the patients still experience unbearable symptoms before death (Ventafridda *et al.*, 1990; cited by Miller, 1992, p.128). Fainsinger says that 16 percent of patients are considered to require sedation because of dramatic pain (Fainsinger, *et.al.*, 1991; cited by Miller, 1992, p.285). Even Cicely Saunders agrees that there are about 10 percent of patients with uncontrollable terminal pain (Humphrey, 1992, p.21). Hence in so far as the hospice does not accept the idea of voluntary active euthanasia, a handful of patients have to suffer before their death. While making great progress in pain control methods for the dying, those who support the hospice ideal should admit the fact that they allow, in the name of God, some patients to suffer from dramatic pain in their terminal stage. Until the hospice succeeds in controlling pain, uncontrollable pain must be left to 'God's hand', because uncontrollable pain will not be the problem of the hospice but of God.

Saunders' attitude to suffering is based upon the Christian idea, so in the end pain is something which we should not control by means such as voluntary active euthanasia, and life and death are also left to God or Nature. The hospice makes every effort to control the patient's pain whether it comes as punishment or for whatever reason, attempting to reduce the weight of the patient's 'cross', but this does not mean that the patient is totally released from his or her cross. Some symptoms are not controllable, and even if physical symptoms are controlled appropriately the patient may next suffer psychological and spiritual pains. While the hospice tries to reduce physical, psychological, and spiritual pains, some of the pain will always remain as 'the cross' of each patient, but it may have to be so because this 'cross' makes cancer patients become 'pilgrims' or makes them identifiable with Christ on the way to his death in the pilgrim-cancer patient metaphor. The hospice is always interested in reducing all kinds of pain of cancer patients, but may not think it right to completely 'destroy' their 'crosses' because they may then no longer be 'pilgrims' to be respected and cared for. So, to some extent, the hospice may value the patient's suffering as his 'cross', and respect the meaning of pain in his life as a mystery, which no one could discern except God, and therefore must not destroy it completely, as with voluntary active euthanasia, even if the pain is unbearable.

The Idea of Voluntary Active Euthanasia

As opposed to the hospice's attitude, the idea of voluntary active euthanasia seems to allow humans to take the initiative in the matter of life, death, and pain, in which the attitude to pain is seen to be much clearer and not mysterious. Pain is considered to be an evil, which must be eliminated, because pain has nothing to do with God but with each individual. The idea of pain merely as evil is different from the hospice's point of view influenced by the Christian idea. The following poem by a member of the Scottish Society expresses the idea of rejecting God as a decision maker eloquently:

Inconsistency

'Thou shalt not kill' -
Except when called to fight
For thine own country's sake,
- Then, 'might is right.'

'Thou shalt not kill.'
No more the hangman's rope
Will terrorists deter -
Let prisons cope.

'Thou shalt not kill' -
Except to take THY life,
When other means have failed.

(Mowat, 1993, p.29)

The Voluntary Euthanasia Society had about 13,000 members in Britain in 1992 and the numbers are growing, while the hospice is trying hard to control the pain of the terminal patient (Japan Society for Dying with Dignity, 1992, p.17). How we connect the increase of the society's membership with the hospice movement depends upon what makes an individual join the society. But the fact that the hospice has not completely succeeded in the relief of some kinds of pain and in accepting all patients who want to stay in the hospice building, may be more or less related to the growing number of the society's members.

Another aspect to consider is that there may be cases where the patient would still request active euthanasia even if all his pain could be dealt with. The patient may insist on the right to choose the time to die or the right to give up his life quickly without 'the cross' or 'pilgrimage'. In this case, the possibility of controlling symptoms, which the hospice tends to insist on, cannot be a sufficient reason for the hospice's disapproval of active euthanasia. So, the hospice may need to give another answer to the paradoxical nature of its philosophy in which it claims to respect the patient's autonomy but at the same time rejects the idea of active euthanasia even if it is the patient's will. We have to remember, however, cancer patients will lose the status of 'pilgrims' or 'penitents' once the hospice philosophy begins to accept the active method of killing them. This is because it will totally destroy the worth of 'the cross' (all sorts of pain experienced by cancer patients) or 'pilgrimage' (the way to the cross), which may be considered to be necessary and valuable in order to gain salvation and to make 'death' meaningful and valuable as Christ's death is in the Christian background of the hospice movement. Once the pilgrim-cancer patient metaphor becomes inapplicable to cancer patients, the implication for cancer and the patient's existence will change and possibly the image of patients may go back again to society's notion of 'a deserted, punished, disrespected sinner'.

3 The Hospice Movement in Japan

Introduction

Japan does not have a long tradition of the hospice movement, which is deeply influenced by Christian ideas, and the concept of the modern hospice movement has been only imported from the West in the 1980s. So, we cannot explore the Japanese hospice and its underlying notions as much as we did for the West, but let us explore firstly how hospice care has begun to be considered and what situation it presently is in; secondly, what sort of difficulty Japan has faced in terms of establishing hospices; and finally, the Japanese attitude to pain and diseases, which will be an important matter when we make a philosophical comparison between the Western and Japanese hospice movements in a later chapter. We use the terms hospice care and palliative care as synonymous in this chapter since Japan has not made a clear distinction between hospice care and palliative care, that is to say, palliative care units in hospitals are often called hospice care units in Japan.

The Japanese Hospice Movement

A History of the Japanese Hospice

As of 1990, more than two hundred thousand Japanese die of cancer annually (Kashiwagi, 1991a, p.92), and it has been the leading cause of death in Japan since 1981 (Kashiwagi, 1991b, p.166). As we will discuss in Part Three on The Doctor-Patient Relationship, Japanese doctors have been more interested in the 'cure' aspect of medicine rather than 'care', and this tendency has led to patients experiencing unnecessary pain caused by aggressive treatments and excessive life-prolongation. The doctor tends to believe in the idea that he should make every effort to save the patient's life even if there is only a one percent possibility of success rather than the idea that he had better give up because there is a ninety-nine percent chance of failure (Yamazaki, 1992, pp.136-37).

However from the 1970s a small group of physicians began to reflect on the cure-oriented approach to medicine and to contemplate the necessity of hospice care (Kashiwagi, 1991b, p.167). According to recent research on Japanese doctors' and nurses' attitudes to hospice care, 40.8 percent of them approve of the hospice movement in Japan (Yamamoto *et al.*, 1990, p.28). Yodogawa Christian Hospital organized a team named 'The Organized Care of the Dying Patient (OCDP)' in 1973, which was the first palliative service in Japan. At the same time some Japanese newspapers reported the work of St Christopher's Hospice in Britain. In 1977 the Japanese Association for Clinical Research on Death and Dying (JARD) was established and by 1990 it had become a large association of more than a thousand members who are mainly nurses and physicians. In 1981, Seirei Hospital in Shizuoka Prefecture built the first Japanese hospice ward inside a hospital (Kashiwagi, 1991b, p.167). In 1993, the Ministry of Health and Welfare had recognised palliative care units in 11 hospitals, but the number of beds in these units were only 231 altogether. By 1997, these numbers had risen somewhat to 35 hospitals and 623 beds (communication to author from Ministry of Health and Welfare).

Difficulties in Developing the Hospice Movement in Japan

Although Japan has begun to reflect on the way of caring for the dying in hospital and to take notice of hospice type care since the 1970s, there are many problems involved in developing hospice care in Japan as follows:

> strongly cure-oriented physicians, patients, and their families;
> a lack of interest in palliative care and pain relief;
> the problem with telling a true diagnosis;
> a lack of carers;
> financial difficulties;
> an unclear concept of the word 'hospice' in the Japanese mind.

Strongly Cure-oriented Physicians, Patients, and Their Families A highly developed National Health Insurance system makes it possible for the Japanese to use health care resources as much as they want until they die. Many Japanese physicians, patients, and their families tend to have the belief that it is good to receive cure-oriented treatments which prolong the patient's life (Hara, 1982, p.115) even in the case of an incurable disease. Even the Showa Emperor stayed in hospital receiving treatment for 111 days before his death, and many Japanese patients asked their doctors to treat them in the way the Emperor was treated, while some Japanese became members of the Japan Society for Dying with Dignity to avoid such excessive life prolongation as was carried out for the Emperor (Oki, 1991, pp.3-4). The modern Japanese, to some extent, still expect cure-oriented medicine in some form and have difficulty in changing this attitude suddenly to concentrate on improving the quality of life of the patient (Nara, 1987, p.97). Japanese hospices are now developing as part of hospital organizations and this leads the Japanese hospice to have the nature of a hospital (Kashiwagi, 1986, p.243); in other words, there is the possibility that caring staff, patients, and their families are likely to seek hospital-type treatment in hospice care.

A Lack of Interest in Palliative Care Japanese doctors and nurses may find it hard to devote themselves only to the incurable since it will cause them a lot of psychological as well as physical stress (Hara, 1982, pp.115-16), while medical professionals normally have not had any support for managing their stress or any psychological education in how to deal with the dying. Another aspect is that death is still seen as a defeat of medical science, which has achieved a great success in curing diseases such as tuberculosis, so doctors still concern themselves more with conquering cancer and death (see Part III). The third aspect is related to difficulties in telling the truth about the diagnosis which we will discuss later. Doctors and nurses do not want to go to see terminally ill cancer patients because they have to hide the true diagnosis from them (Yamazaki, 1992, p.144). Considering these three dimensions, we can easily see why very few medical professionals pursue an interest in palliative care.

One of the most crucial purposes of Western hospice care has been to control the pain of cancer patients. Also in Japan, since the publication of 'Cancer Pain Relief' published by the World Health Organization (WHO), doctors and nurses have begun to be interested in pain control over the past few years (Kashiwagi, 1991b, p.168). But morphine is still not sufficiently given for controlling terminal cancer pain because of the concern that the patient might become dependent upon the drug (Oki, 1991, p.81); the bad image of morphine (Yamazaki, 1992, p.144) as 'a medicine for death'; complex law procedures in which doctors have to submit pages of documents to use the drug; and also because of the Japanese attitude to pain, which tends to encourage patients to bear pain (Naito, 1992, p.170). Hospice care in Japan tends to be expected to develop inside hospitals, but pain control, one of the first priorities in the hospice philosophy, may not be easy since Japanese hospitals do not yet seem to be keen on using drugs like morphine for terminal cancer patients.

The Problem with Telling the Truth about the Diagnosis   Only 16.9 percent of Japanese physicians have ever told their patients of a diagnosis of cancer (Sakari, 1980, p.50, cited by Nagata, 1982, p.5). Doctors may reveal the diagnosis to the family but usually not to the patient himself. Many Japanese patients die, not knowing or questioning the true nature of their disease (Kashiwagi, 1991a, p.85, p.169). In eight Japanese palliative care units, only 49 percent of patients knew the true diagnosis. Nagata explores conditions in which the doctor may tell the true diagnosis to the patient as follows:

> (i) after a good relationship between the doctor and the patient (including the family) is established;
> (ii) the patient has a strong sense of self or faith without becoming desperate which enables him or her to become a member of the curing team after the diagnosis and to have the ability to achieve his or her social role and responsibility;
> (iii) the patient has supportive family or friends;
> (iv) the patient's cancer is still at the early stage or is predicted to be recognized by himself even if he or she is not told;
> (v) the patient can be supported by a health care team who continue to brush up their attitudes towards life and death (e.g. The Balint Group[1]) and can give hope to the patient. (Nagata, 1982, p.8; translated by myself)

We discover at least two important features of Japanese medicine from the above. Firstly, it seems that the decision maker for 'truth telling' is not considered to be the patient or his or her family but someone else, usually a doctor, who makes a judgment in regard to the five conditions; and secondly, the patient's individual 'rights' and 'autonomy' are not taken seriously. Meeting all five requirements must be difficult and that means

---

[1] The Balint Group was established by Michael Balint, a medical doctor as well as a psychoanalyst, who worked in London. He developed a method of medical interview which emphasized a certain sort of 'listening' to patients and could discover psychosocial causes hidden behind patients' ordinary physical symptoms by looking at patients in a holistic way. For the purpose of teaching this way of approaching patients to GPs in London, the Balint Group was formed around the end of the 1930s (Ikemi, 1988, p.257).

the truth generally will be hidden from the patient, though the requirements would not be a sufficient basis for deciding about the disclosure if the patient's rights and autonomy were emphasized as in the West.

If the majority of Japanese incurable cancer patients knew that they had got an incurable disease, they might be able to choose hospice care rather than continuing with curative treatments. In fact, however, the patient does not know the truth usually, so it is often the family who want the patient to receive hospice care (Kashiwagi, 1991a, p.91). Without the patients' own awareness of the need for hospice-type care, there may be limitations to developing it in the same way as the West does, and without 'truth telling' it is hard to strengthen the awareness.

Lack of Carers In its emphasis on care-centred medicine in hospice care, the essential nature of palliative care stresses nursing and nurses as having an important role. However, Japan has had a serious problem with both a shortage and the low social status of nurses. Currently there are eighty thousand nurses in Japan and there is a shortage of about fifty thousand nurses. Every year, fifty-five thousand nurses are newly employed but at the same time about forty thousand nurses give up their jobs. So Japan has to suffer continuously from a shortage of nursing labour. As a result, nurses are forced to work extremely hard and cannot provide a good quality of nursing for each of their patients (Sawada, 1992, p.1).

The reasons for the shortage of nurses and the increase in nurses giving up their jobs come from various sources. The first is, as mentioned, overwork: 60 percent of Japanese nurses complain about problems with their health such as eye strain, headache, a stiff neck and shoulder, chronic physical and mental fatigue, depression, etc. In this condition, nurses may find it hard and stressful to work with incurable cancer patients, who physically and psychologically need special treatments. Secondly, we have to think about the dramatic increase of hospital beds after the Second World War, from which the problem of nursing labour shortage began. The third is nurses' dissatisfaction with the quality of their jobs in physician-centred Japanese hospitals, in which nurses work merely as assistants to physicians and cannot achieve the true nature of nursing, that is, caring for their patients. Nurses are low in Japanese social hierarchies, and they are regarded not as specialists but as nothing more than doctors' maids. To some extent, a long Japanese history of social inequality between men and women may be related to nurses' low status. Moreover, one can become a nurse without graduating from university and a person's educational background is very important in Japan where forty percent of the young population go to universities (Sawada, 1992, pp.2-5).

The nature of hospice care is likely to imply a focus on nursing, so the role of nurses should be taken seriously, but the shortage of nurses makes it difficult. And even if there were enough nurses who were interested in hospice care, their low social position in physician-oriented hospitals would not allow them to be in a leading position in the Japanese hospice movement (Kashiwagi, 1991b, p.168), which tends to be developed inside hospitals. Additionally, a lack of caring staff is compounded by a lack of voluntary workers since they are not welcomed by hospitals (Hara, 1982, p.115).

Financial Difficulty The Japanese health care service is based upon a scheme started in 1961, which gives health care insurance to every individual; the doctor's freedom of private practice through a simple process; a reimbursement based mainly upon a 'fees for service (payment by results) system' (Kashiwagi, 1991b, p.165). This encourages Japanese self-contained hospitals to prolong their hospitalization unnecessarily, give medication or injections, and provide examinations, because otherwise they could not maintain themselves financially.

In 1990, the Japanese Government established special charges for hospitalization in the palliative care units of the eleven hospitals recognised by the Welfare Ministry. Through this special support, the hospitals could receive 30,000 yen (£176; £1 = 170yen) a day for each patient staying on the palliative care ward, which was not 'fees for service' but the amount to be paid regardless of the actual cost (Kashiwagi, 1993). Although this new special charge has helped the eleven hospitals financially as they no longer need to unnecessarily increase the number of services for patients, the government gives such support only to those hospitals which can meet certain requirements (Kashiwagi, 1991b, p.168), which many other hospitals may not be able to satisfy easily. It is unrealistic to think that all the two hundred thousand patients dying of cancer every year can be treated in the eleven hospice care units alone, 231 beds being the total number of beds in palliative care units altogether. The financial barrier is an important factor also in the difficulty there is in establishing hospices outside hospitals in Japan.

An Unclear Concept of the Word 'Hospice' in the Japanese Mind Japan has not had the historical background of the hospice movement as the West has since medieval times, and hospice care tends to occur inside hospitals, so the Japanese may find it difficult to have the image of the word 'hospice' as 'a house for pilgrims'. In other words, the metaphorical connection between cancer patients and medieval pilgrims, which has been discussed in Chapter 2, does not exist in Japan. Furthermore, because a true diagnosis is normally told to the family but not to the patient himself, and the family (rather than the patient himself) wants the patient to receive hospice care, the Japanese concept of the term 'hospice' or 'hospice care' will be dissimilar to the Western one. Without appreciating this and redefining the word 'hospice' for the Japanese medical and social environment, the word 'hospice' remains unclear in the Japanese mind and hospice care may not be easily popularized. Even if Japanese medicine introduces the Western concept of 'hospice' but ignores the differences, it may cause a lot of problems, as we will discuss in later chapters.

The Image of the Cancer Patient

The Idea of Disease as 'Dirt' and 'Impurity'

Although we have not got any relevant material which explores particularly the Japanese image of cancer or cancer patients directly, let us consider it through an investigation of the Japanese attitude to disease in relation to the understanding of disease as 'dirt' or 'impurity'. Japanese children are taught to take their shoes off and wash their hands when they come into their home from the outside. The idea is that there are 'dirts' and germs outside so one must take one's shoes off in order to avoid getting dirt from the outside into the clean inside. In Japanese baby language 'bacchi' (dirty) is an important word taught to small children by their parents who point out things that are thought to be dirty and ought not to be touched (Ohnuki-Tierney, 1984, pp.21-26).

It is, therefore, not surprising that the hospital, as a house full of those with diseases is seen as one of the dirtiest places in the Japanese mind. At the National Institute for Cancer Research, all the books returned by patients are normally wiped with alcohol (Inoue, 1981; cited by Ohnuki-Tierney, 1984, p.30), and here we can see that there is the idea of cancer as something 'dirty' or 'impure', which may be transmitted from the patients to others, though cancer is not contagious (Ohnuki-

Tierney, 1984, pp.27-30). This symbolic idea of the 'impurity of disease' has been found through the centuries in Japan. According to the Norito (AD 967), which is a book of Shinto prayers to the Gods, 'impurity' is regarded as the greatest sin of all and killing or handling corpses, and getting diseases are considered as sins of impurity (Philippi, 1959, p.46; cited by Ohnuki-Tierney, 1984, p.36). Even in contemporary Japan, when one comes back from a funeral, where the person has spent time with a corpse, his family bring salt to sprinkle over him before he enters the house (p.25).

Individual Responsibility for Disease

In the Japanese idea of 'dirt' and 'impurity', they come from 'outside' the person, and the person may be a passive victim of the 'dirt' or 'impurity' of disease, so he or she may not have to take much responsibility for their diseased condition. The strong tradition of 'fatalism' under the Buddhist influence could explain this attitude to disease, where the Japanese tend to accept disease and death as one's own fate, since they recognise disease and death as a part of the supernatural and encompassing universe (Ishiwata and Sakai, 1994, p.63). In the Shinto tradition, the cause of disease has been understood as the departed soul (Nakajima, 1988, p.2; cited by Ishiwata and Sakai, 1994, p.63), and in this interpretation disease is not likely to be the fault of the person who lost his or her soul. Moreover, the Japanese people are often proud of having a delicate and weak body, which can easily become diseased (Caudill, 1976, p.162; cited by Ohnuki-Tierney, 1984, p.52). To be delicate in body and mind means to be sensitive and this sensitivity relates to the image of intellectuals or academics, while the Japanese word 'mushinkei (no nerves or sensitivity)' is used for a person who is insensitive in body as well as mind and even stupid. We can see a paradox here, in which disease is 'impurity' and 'sin', but, at the same time, the weakness of the human's mind and body in getting them seems to be thought of as being sensitive and intelligent. This paradox leads to the fact that the Japanese are quite open about their own illness (Ohnuki-Tierney, 1984, pp.52-60).

Attitude to Happiness

We may be able to explain this paradox by the Japanese attitude to happiness. Minami observes that, in contrast to foreigners, the Japanese people tend to be reluctant about expressing happiness and this is deeply related to the Japanese emphasis on the virtue of enduring unhappiness. This hesitation about happiness can be found in the Japanese tendency of not using the word 'happiness' in their daily conversation, while the Japanese language is rich in vocabulary for expressing 'unhappiness', 'hardship', and 'difficulty'. The noun 'tears', the verb 'cry', and the adjectives 'distressing', 'sorrowful', and 'lonesome' are frequently used in Japanese popular songs. Considering this, the Japanese seem to think about unhappiness in relation to their own lives oftener than happiness (Minami, 1971, pp.34-49).

There has always been the idea in Japanese history: 'Near satisfaction is unsatisfactory, but complete satisfaction is hazardous' (Minami, 1971, pp.34-49). For example, Kaibara Ekiken wrote *Kadokun (Introduction to a family way of life)* in 1711 and said in this book:

> There is a limit to a man's wealth, but there is no limit to his avarice. If he indulges himself in avarice, his wealth will, without fail, be depleted. ... If he acts as he pleases, forgetting the limit to his wealth, no matter how rich he may be he will use up all wealth ... . (Ekiken, 1711; cited by Minami, 1971, p.36)

Also, Hayashi Razan, a Confucian scholar taught in *Shunkansho (Treatise on five virtues)*:

> If you indulge your desires, you will certainly ruin yourself in the future. If you give full swing to your inclinations, you will without fail destroy yourself. If you go to extreme in seeking pleasures, you will encounter sorrow in the end. If you restrict yourself, you will be able to avoid catastrophe ... (Razan, 1629; quoted by Minami, 1971, p.36)

The main idea underlying these two descriptions is that we should not seek happiness or pleasure too much but restrict them. Japanese people may feel guilty if they are completely happy and almost prefer imperfection in their life, where individuals will not get what they want but lose what they do not. The essential Japanese perspective on life might be called 'fatalism' and 'nihilism'. The former is the idea that the happiness or unhappiness of humans is a destiny brought by Karma in relation to a previous life as Buddhism teaches, and the latter emphasizes that in this world everything is impermanent and one can discover an absolute being only by denying happiness (Minami, 1971, pp.43-52). 'Fatalism' and 'nihilism' have survived through centuries, and we could say that pain and hardship are, to some extent, necessary for the Japanese idea of happiness; in other words, you are not allowed to become happy unless you have had pain and hardship, whether physically or mentally.

Coming back to the Japanese attitude to disease, they seem to be proud of having pain or hardship caused by their disease. Disease is caused by impurity and dirt so may be seen as a 'sin', but 'sin' may be necessary for the Japanese idea of happiness. The paradoxical way, in which Japanese people make a great effort to avoid 'dirt' in their daily life, while they are also proud of being ill through acquiring 'dirt', might be interpreted through the idea that both avoiding 'dirt' or being ill by acquiring 'dirt' are a sort of evidence of their sensitive and delicate nature. You try to 'purify' 'dirt' from the outside by washing your hands and taking your shoes off because you are sensitive and delicate enough to be involved. And in the end you may become ill but the fact that you as 'a sensitive person' get 'the impurity' of disease identifies you as 'pure' and 'sensitive'. If we put the word 'sin' instead of 'disease' or 'impurity', we may say that a sensitive person always 'purifying' herself sometimes has to shoulder the burden of 'sin' for which she is not responsible. This misfortune and sadness may make her existence special and even heroic. So the Japanese people keep saying that they have got certain diseases by calling them 'jibyo (my disease)' (Ohnuki-Tierney, 1984, p.53), in order to show, unconsciously in most cases, that they are 'sensitive, intelligent, and unfortunate beings' who have to suffer from illness (impurity) despite their 'purity'. Hence people may want to think themselves weak and sensitive. It is sad to get disease despite the fact that you are always pure or try to make the effort to be so, and it is unfortunate that a 'pure' person is attacked by disease, but it makes your existence special. The Japanese idea of happiness seems to be deeply related to this 'sadness' and 'misfortune', where you are happy when you are an object of compassion and have a certain image of sadness and misfortune.

In the case of cancer, however, the Japanese mind may interpret it differently from the way they do for any other disease. One big difference is that people do not openly discuss cancer. Ohnuki-Tierney points out that the Japanese attitude towards cancer is very similar to the attitude of Western people (p.61) as described in Chapter 2, which includes an individual responsibility for the disease as a sin within the person. But we would not entirely agree with this, considering the very different attitudes to death between the West and Japan which we will analyze in a later chapter, and also the Japanese image of cancer as a disease coming from outside, as shown earlier by the fact that books borrowed by cancer patients are wiped with alcohol though cancer is not contagious.

The Japanese may also consider that 'cancer dirt' comes not only from the outside but also from the inside of the patient if we accept Ohnuki-Tierney's point of view. If there is any room in the Japanese mind for individual responsibility for cancer, it might be distinguished from other diseases. Nevertheless, the Japanese patient does not have to take the responsibility because of the customary lack of disclosure of the diagnosis; in other words, the patient does not have to know his 'sinfulness' but the people surrounding him shoulder his 'sins' on his behalf. We may be able to think about death in the same way; that is to say, a diagnosis of cancer tends to imply death even if it is curable and individual responsibility for death is reduced by non-disclosure, while carers and the patient's family shoulder the burden of death. Therefore, individual responsibility for cancer is even more reduced compared to other diseases, whether 'impurity' and 'sin' are considered to come from inside or outside the person.

4 A Comparison of Japanese and Western Hospice Movements

Similarities

Infantilization of the Patient

There might be a possibility that both the Western and the Japanese hospice create the dependency of the patient since the hospice is likely to offer a uniform pathway to death. If Western patients are metaphorically 'pilgrims' on the way to salvation, it is not the patient who provides the hospice-pilgrimage image but the hospice philosophy itself. Prima facie, the Western hospice philosophy respects the patient's individual rights and autonomy, but the patient is expected to live the hospice community life, which is already set up, and this may lead to the process of infantilization of the patient. The patient may be passively put into the pilgrim-cancer patient metaphor once they are admitted into hospice care, and be forced to be a hero or heroine of the drama of 'pilgrimage'. On the other hand, Japanese cancer patients may also be infantilized since they are likely to be accepted into hospice care units without knowing the nature of their disease unless their families' will it. Their lives are highly dependent upon the decision-making of others such as doctors, nurses, and relatives. Cancer patients do not have to take any individual responsibility for their diseases even if the disease could raise the idea of guilt inside the person, because they are normally not told the diagnosis. So, both the Western and the Japanese hospice have the inherent ability to infantilize dying cancer patients.

A Perspective on Pain

Secondly, let us discuss some similarities between the Western and the Japanese hospice movements in relation to their attitudes to pain and suffering. The modern hospice began with a concern about cancer patients' pain during the dying process both in the West and Japan. This must be considered together with the modern reflection and re-examination of the way the dying are treated in hospitals, as we have already mentioned in previous chapters.   But the first priority of the hospice has always been pain control; in other words, the modern hospice movement might not have occurred without the reality that many dying cancer patients have suffered from cure-centred aggressive and dehumanized treatments, which prolong their lives and agony needlessly. The West and Japan are similar, therefore, in the fact that the underlying aim behind the rise of the hospice movement for the dying, particularly for incurable cancer patients, is to control patients' pain.

Despite such a strong emphasis on symptom-control, the Western hospice has, on the other hand, been against voluntary active euthanasia even though some ten percent of terminal cancer pain is considered to be uncontrollable.   As we have seen in Chapter 2, the hospice philosophy with its strong Christian background might regard such pain as a mystery and respect the profound meaning of 'the cross' and the patient's 'pilgrimage'.   In Christianity, an individual is supposed to carry his or her own cross, and this itself will be the way to salvation: ' . . . if any man will come after me, let him deny himself, and take up his own cross, and follow me' (Matthew 16: 24).   While the hospice makes every effort to reduce the patient's pain, whether physical or psychological, it does not destroy his 'cross' totally but helps him to shoulder it.   This Christian attitude to pain and suffering may correspond to the Japanese attitude to happiness.   The Japanese perspective on happiness is likely to be found in the pursuit of imperfectionism (Chapter 3), in which pain and hardship are, to some extent, necessary for the Japanese idea of happiness; in other words, we cannot be easily made happy without having had some pain. Interestingly, this reminds us of the Sermon on the Mount in the New Testament:

> Blessed are they that mourn: for they shall be comforted; (Matthew 5: 4)
> Blessed are they which do hunger and thirst after righteousness: for they shall be filled; (6)
> Blessed are they which are persecuted for righteousness' sake: for their's is the kingdom of heaven. (10)

We may not want to be in the situation where we mourn losing our loved ones, nor to live in a society full of injustice, where we thirst after righteousness, nor be persecuted for righteousness' sake, but Jesus says that we are happy then.   Jesus even teaches (Luke 6: 24-25):

> But woe unto you that are rich! For ye have received your consolation.

Woe unto you that are full! for ye shall hunger.
Woe unto you that laugh now! for ye shall mourn and weep.

We have no intention of giving a theological account of these quotations, but let us consider them from the aspect of 'the cross'. The reason that those who mourn, thirst, and are persecuted are happy may be because they are in a way shouldering their cross because of the pains involved in their situations.   To carry one's own cross is a crucial theme in Christianity since Jesus himself suggested it to his followers, and this is the only way to gain salvation.   When we are in pain of some kind and accept it with courage and love, Christianity may say that we are walking towards God and his salvation, so this may bring Christian happiness more than anything else.   Although it may be easier for someone to avoid all the pain of persecution or not thirst after righteousness through his cowardice, this means to throw away his cross and turn away from God in the end, so he may be unhappy in Jesus' eyes even if he can laugh or be full now.   Another way of thinking about Jesus' words is from the view that both pain and pleasure in this life will not last forever. If we are laughing now, we will mourn and cry in the future, but if we mourn now, we will be comforted and laugh again ... and if we laugh again, we will have to mourn and cry again in the future.   So neither pain nor pleasure lasts forever in this life.   This idea reminds us of the Buddhist notion that everything is impermanent, and seems to be related to the Japanese attitude to happiness and unhappiness.

Not only has Japan found happiness in imperfection or in pain and suffering, but also the West with its Christian tradition has valued the meaning of pain and suffering in order to discover and gain a true happiness.   Therefore, although one of the reasons for the difficulty in developing the hospice in Japan is (as seen in Chapter 3) its attitude to pain, which encourages the patient to bear with his pain, the Japanese perspective on pain is not totally alien to the Western hospice's attitude to pain and suffering which follows the Christian interpretation.

Bias to Cancer Patients

The third important similarity is that hospices are most likely to admit patients dying of cancer rather than of any other diseases. We have suggested several reasons for the Western hospice's particular interest in cancer patients, who suit hospice-type care (Chapter 2).   At least two physical reasons were considered: firstly, many people die of cancer with severe chronic pain and the modern hospice movement began with the purpose of giving special attention to conquering their pain; secondly, the nature of cancer is particularly suitable for hospice type care as we explored in Chapter 2. As to Japanese hospices, it seems to be taken for granted that the object of hospice care is cancer patients, as we tend to find that research on Japanese hospices does not question this. This is understandable considering the fact that Japan has taken the idea of the hospice from the Western hospice movement, which has always had a special focus on cancer, though the concept of hospice is still unclear in the Japanese mind. The hospice's particular concentration on cancer patients could prevent the idea of hospice care becoming a philosophy of care in general. The West and Japan will continue to have this problem as long as hospices are very much cancer patient-biased (except for a few Western hospices for AIDS patients, which have been established in recent years).

Differences

Infantilization

There are many differences between the Western and the Japanese hospice movements, but the most crucial of all may be the fact that Japanese patients are not like 'pilgrims' but 'babies', and that Western cancer patients may be in the process of infantilization but can never be likened to 'babies'. In an ordinary Japanese life, important decisions in an individual's life are normally made by or with his family or the community. This is reflected also in the medical sphere, where all medical decision-making depends upon doctors and families. In the case of incurable cancer patients, however, the dependency is even stronger mainly because of a lack of disclosure of the diagnosis, so that patients do not have to take any responsibility for their disease. So Japanese cancer patients become like babies, who are passively looked after by people surrounding them, and are not likely to (be able to) make decisions on their own.

Despite the fact that there is a degree of infantilization, dying cancer patients in the West are not like 'babies' even in the hospice, since within the setting of the pilgrim-cancer patient metaphor they are still treated as responsible adults supposed to shoulder their cross of pain as their own responsibility. No matter how much the hospice gives support to patients to carry on their own pilgrimages with their crosses, it cannot destroy the cross completely but encourages patients to walk on their own. Christianity, which provides the strong background behind the pilgrim-cancer patient metaphor, respects individuality and the notion of individual responsibility for one's own life by one's own decision, because God has a purpose for each person's life individually. Therefore, while the Western hospice may infantilize cancer patients forcing them to become involved with the pilgrim-cancer patient metaphor, it cannot treat them as babies as part of its Christian philosophy. But Japanese cancer 'babies' cannot be 'pilgrims' like Western patients, and do not walk on their feet nor know clearly where they are going to (death) nor in what sort of way (cancer).

The difference between the West and Japan in the matter of individual responsibility of a patient for his own life and disease can also be considered together with 'the purification of threefold guilt', which is one of the strengths of the pilgrim-cancer patient metaphor. In Japan, the guilt is twofold (the guilt of doctors and the families) because patients are protected from all punitive connotations of cancer, even if there were any, by their families and carers who hide the diagnosis. Because of this lack of disclosure, the guilt of the doctor and the family may partly remain, though there may be a degree of change in the roles for the patient, the family, and the doctor in the Japanese hospice. Japanese doctors and families withhold the truth from their consideration that it is the best for the patient, but may continue to feel guilty about their deception.

Perspectives on Pain

We have already discussed that the perspective on pain and suffering is in a sense similar between the West and Japan, both of which respect the meaning of pain in terms of gaining true happiness, but we also need to bring out a difference in how Western and Japanese people behave when facing pain. If it is correct to say that the Japanese tend to accept pain as something deriving from Nature, fate, or karma as we will consider in Chapter 6. Their main attitude is to wait rather passively for the time of pleasure to arrive naturally or to entrust their pain to other people, who may find a way of destroying the pain. Because nothing is permanent, they tend to passively accept that the time for pain as well as the time for pleasure should be left to come naturally.

On the other hand, the Christian idea of carrying one's own cross may imply a more active attitude to pain and suffering, in which an individual does not just give up and accept the painful condition as fate but shoulders his own cross of pain by himself and follows Christ so that he can gain salvation, a true happiness. Walking when shouldering a cross to gain true happiness entails an active attitude compared to accepting one's own destiny and waiting for the good times to come.

The Bias to Cancer Patients in Hospices

Not all dying people can be 'pilgrims' in the Western hospice and 'babies' in the Japanese hospice, but only cancer patients are entitled to be 'pilgrims' or 'babies'. We have discovered that this is one of the similarities between the Western and the Japanese hospice movements. Although the Western and the Japanese hospice are similar in physical aspects as explained in Seale's research (see Chapter 2), they need to be separated in philosophical respects with regard to the different nature of the pilgrim-cancer patient metaphor and the baby-cancer patient metaphor. In the pilgrim-cancer patient metaphor, we can find religious reasons which make cancer patients particularly appropriate to the metaphor of 'pilgrimage', since cancer tends to have a strong punitive connotation in the West. Cancer patients may be seen as 'deserted strangers', while their disease itself and the topic of death are taboo in modern Western society, where the image of cancer patients covers the ideas of sin, pilgrimage and the cross which are involved in the metaphor. However, the Japanese baby-cancer patient metaphor, which implies the patient's passivity, could not coexist with the Western pilgrim-cancer patient metaphor in the end, because it implies the patient's individual responsibility for and active attitude to his 'cross' in his 'pilgrimage'. So in Japan there seems to be no significant religious implication by which cancer patients particularly attract hospice care.

The Nature of the Term 'Hospice' in Relation to Christianity

As the term 'hospice' has a strong Christian tradition in the West, Seirei hospital, which established the first hospice ward in Japan is, in fact, a Christian hospital, and about half of the government-acknowledged palliative care units belong to Christian hospitals. This may be because Christian hospitals in Japan accept the idea of the Western hospice with its Christian philosophy more easily than other secular hospitals could. However, the Christian hospice care wards in Japan have to face complicated cross-cultural and religious issues. For example, as previously described, Japanese cancer patients in hospices are not seen as 'pilgrims' but as 'babies'. The Christian hospice philosophy may not approve of dying cancer patients being 'babies', but may encourage them to be adults capable of pilgrimages within the metaphorical setting. Preparation for death and completion of life as a 'pilgrimage' with the cross of pain and suffering are crucial, where individual responsibility for life is essential. Not to take responsibility, thus becoming a baby, means to reject the cross. Japanese Christian hospices, therefore, may face a dilemma between recognising 'cancer pilgrims' or 'cancer babies' in the two metaphors.

While the West has begun to develop palliative care in hospitals independently from the hospice organization and its religious connotation, with regard to Japanese secular hospitals having hospice care units, we are not certain how they define the term 'hospice' and distinguish or identify 'hospice wards' from/with 'palliative care units'. We may say that in the West what is going on in hospices is a form of palliative care, but we would not say that palliative care in hospitals is the same as hospice care, because the former do not just give palliative care but can be a religious form of palliative care which involves the pilgrim-cancer patient metaphor. Hence it is almost impossible to use the term 'hospice' in total isolation from the metaphor, but palliative care does not imply such a metaphor or religious meaning. In some Japanese medical journals, palliative care and hospice care are treated as the same, and Japanese books and articles are often written about the hospice beginning with the origin of the term ('a house for pilgrims') in a positive and accepting manner. We can even find an expression like 'There may be a future when we can live without worries about death because of the existence of the hospice' (Yamazaki, 1993, pp.358-62; translated by myself).

But the Japanese do not seem to have a clear definition of 'hospice', and they may not be able to use the term in the same way when they have clarified and understood its religious connotation which relates to the pilgrim-cancer patient metaphor, and is not applicable to Japanese cancer 'babies'. Thus, both Christian and non-Christian hospices in Japan are predicted to suffer from a conceptual gap between 'cancer pilgrims' and 'cancer babies' in connection with their attitude to death, human relationships, individual rights, and autonomy, as long as they use the word 'hospice'.

The Risk of Creating a Certain Ideal Way of Death

We saw in Chapter 2 that Western hospices may be in danger of creating a certain ideal way of death and dying as if the hospice is the only way for dying cancer patients, due to their confusion between the notion of 'care-only' in the medieval hospice and 'care-centred' in the modern hospice. Japanese hospices may also place their 'faith' in a certain way of death and dying represented only by themselves, but the situation is more complicated than in the West. This is because the Japanese try to bring Western ideas about the hospice to Japanese cancer patients regardless of the dilemma between 'cancer pilgrims' and 'cancer babies', or of the difficulty in applying the Western hospice philosophy, with its strong Christian background, to Japanese people.

The Japanese seem to believe that they have imported the idea of the Western hospice, but in reality the Japanese hospice is not always consistent with the Western hospice ideals as shown above. If the Japanese have begun to feel that hospice care is the only way for dying cancer patients despite the unclear notion of the Japanese hospice which the dilemmas outlined raise, there may be serious problems. That is because Japanese 'cancer babies' are suddenly asked to become independent adults expected to make a pilgrimage on their own, or to remain 'babies' even if they want to die their own death knowing the nature of their disease and making medical decisions more independently from their families and carers. Moreover, Japanese cancer patients can more easily be forced to accept a certain ideal way of death and dying organized by the hospice than Western cancer patients, as they are passive as well as dependent 'babies'.

Hospices as a Reaction against Hospitals and the Idea of Voluntary Active Euthanasia

Japanese hospice care tends to develop inside hospitals due to financial difficulties in establishing buildings independently from hospitals, and this makes it difficult for the Japanese to have the image of the hospice as 'a house for pilgrims'. The Western hospice movement reflects a strong reaction against the modern image of dehumanized hospitalization and also the idea of voluntary active euthanasia, and has established hospice buildings outside hospitals. So, to some extent, Western hospices can more easily establish their own ideals which differ from or are against those of hospitals. Japanese hospices inside hospital buildings may find it hard to realize their dreams and ideals, since it is not realistic that the method of care in hospice wards can go against that of other wards in the same building; in other words, the Japanese hospice philosophy may not be able to isolate itself completely from the way of hospitals.

With regard to the pilgrim-cancer patient and the baby-cancer patient metaphor, the former has a moral implication which changes the moral status of cancer patients from deserted, punished and disrespected sinners into innocent pilgrims or penitents, but the latter does not contain such moral values. The moral connotation involved in the Western metaphor also encourages the hospice (where cancer patients are treated as innocent 'pilgrims') to react strongly against the hospital (where they are treated as 'sinners'), but the Japanese hospice (where 'babies' are) is prevented from becoming a reaction against the hospital (where 'dependent adults' are) because there is no serious moral difference between someone already supposed to be dependent upon others in the culture and someone becoming even more dependent like babies in hospice care.

As to voluntary euthanasia, the current Japanese hospice is not considered to be a reaction against it, because the Japan Society for Dying with Dignity does not encourage any active means of letting an individual die but focuses on spreading Living Wills through the country, and emphasizes the maximization of pain control even if it may shorten an individual's life (which some people would describe as passive euthanasia), and the refusal of life-prolongation in the case of incurable diseases and the persistent vegetative state. These are measures which do not challenge the hospice ideals which accept this form of passive euthanasia in its stress on pain control. But many Western voluntary euthanasia movements insist not only on such passive measures but also on the patient's right to die by the use of active methods even in cases where patients do not have any unendurable pain, so the Western hospice represents a reaction against voluntary euthanasia.

PART II
ATTITUDES TO DEATH AND DYING AND THE HOSPICE MOVEMENT

5 The Western Attitude to Death and Dying

Introduction

In the West the attitude to death has changed over the past centuries, and it seems to be deeply related particularly to the rise of individualism, the Enlightenment, and de-Christianization. Changes in this theme reflect the art of people's living from one age to another, and are mirrored in the hospice movement, which has been seen as an important alternative for the care of the dying, especially for cancer patients, cancer being one of the most common causes of death in the modern Western world. For the purpose of discovering the relationship between the attitudes to death and dying and the hospice movement, this chapter is divided into two parts: in the first section, we will look at how the Western attitude to death and dying has changed in past centuries, and in the second section we will consider the attitude to death and dying together with the nature of the hospice movement.

The History of the Western Attitude to Death and Dying

From the Early Christian Era until the Twelfth Century

Aries uses the expression 'Tamed Death' for the attitude to death from the time of the early Christian era until about the twelfth century, in which death was a familiar event in people's daily life (Aries, 1974, p.2, p.55). Death was understood as a predictable event for each individual as Aries illustrates from the story of the Round Table and the poems about Tristan. Both King Ban in the story of the Round Table and the poems about Tristan predict that their death will arrive soon, as shown in their words. In the Story of the Round Table King Ban says 'O Lord God ... help me, for I see and I know that my end has come'; and in the poems about Tristan, 'Tristan, wounded by a poisoned weapon, 'felt his life spilling out'. He knew that he was about to die' (Aries, 1981, pp.5-6).

The dying person could predict his or her death as it became close and so prepare for it (Aries, 1974, p.7). There were three most important moments in this ceremony: 'the dying man's acceptance of his active role in death (1), the scene of the farewells (2), the scene of mourning (3)' (Aries, 1981, p.603) The person could organize his own public death ritual and know how it would proceed (Aries, 1974, p.11). Death was not an act of an individual but of the community, so the purpose of the death ritual which included (1) to (3) was symbolically to cement the individual's solidarity with his family and community. The community bond would be partly and temporarily destroyed by the death of their members, because an individual's life had an important meaning for the strength or the social structure of the community and for their future (Aries, 1981, p.603).

In the Christian tradition, physical death is not believed to be the end of life but is considered to lead the dead to a waiting period before the resurrection of the body at the end of the world (Aries, 1981, p.604). Because of the belief in the resurrection of the dead body, cremation was not accepted until the modern period (Aries, 1974, p.91). As death was near and familiar to the society, the dying were not isolated from the living but one individual's death and the bereavement of the family after his or her death involved the whole community (Aries, 1974, pp.13-14). This involvement might explain one of the important reasons why death was not the object of fear at that time. Another crucial reason was the faith in the resurrection, which enabled people to accept death as the order of nature which did not elicit any denial or great fear.

From the Twelfth until the Fourteenth Century

The twelfth century is considered as the time of the emergence of individualism which began with the humanism movement, in which it became possible for people to express their thoughts in the Latin language (Morris, 1972, p.9). That is to say, people in the West became more aware of their existence as individuals and their own unique self distinguished from their occupation of a social role (Baumeister, 1986; cited by Kearl, 1989, p.37). Aries calls this period the time of 'one's own death', which was recognised by people who were awakened to their existence as individuals. The idea of individualism is interestingly linked with the scenes expressed on tombstones, and can be differentiated from those in previous centuries. On the tomb of Bishop Agilbert of about 680, an image was drawn which was inspired by Christ in the Apocalypse returning at the end of the world, but there was no place for representing individual responsibility in the counting of good and bad deeds.

Unlike the former centuries, tombstones from the twelfth century began to have a new image under the portrayal of Christ, which was inspired by the book of Matthew. This showed the resurrection of the dead; the separation of the just and the unjust; the Last Judgment; and the weighing of souls by the archangel Michael (Aries, 1974, pp.27-31). While the Judgment scene had not been expressed in the early Christian period, each individual now had to take individual responsibility for his or her deeds in life. In the thirteenth century, two acts were particularly emphasized, one was the weighing of souls and another, the intercession of the Virgin Mary and St. John. In the weighing of souls, good and bad deeds were written in a book. From the end of the fifteenth to the beginning of the sixteenth century, this book finally became an individual report book, which was hung from the dead person's neck (Aries, 1974, pp.31-32).

Death began to be something to be feared from the twelfth century, firstly because of the beginning of the recognition of an individual self, which made people more aware of the Last Judgment for each of themselves, and secondly because of a heightened awareness of death from epidemics and plagues (Kearl, 1989, p.36) most notably the Black Death in the middle of the fourteenth century.

From the Fifteenth to the Seventeenth Century

In this period death was no longer a phenomenon shared by the whole society but something faced and dealt with by the person alone. 'Ars Morrendi', which was a manual on the art of dying, was published and became a best-seller during the fifteenth and the sixteenth centuries. This attempted to revive the traditional image of death from early Christian times. At the end of the fifteenth century, death began to be presented as an erotic image. Writings from the sixteenth to the eighteenth centuries were interested in connecting the theme of death (Thanatos) with love (Eros). For example, in Bernini's portrait of the spiritual union of St Theresa of Avila with God, the anguish of her death and an orgasmic trance were expressed together. A parallel was drawn between death and the sexual act, as death began to be understood as a phenomenon which cuts people off from their rational daily lives (Aries, 1974, pp.34-57). Through the influence of Romanticism from the seventeenth century, cemeteries contained angels 'with increasing hope in a desirable immortality and Romantic faith in the perfectibility of man', and 'there was a concurrent change from skeletal images to portrayals of winged cherubs on the gravestones' (Kearl, 1989, pp.53-54).

From the Eighteenth to the Nineteenth Century

From the eighteenth century, a new implication was given to death, by dramatizing it. Individuals became more interested in the death of other persons than that of themselves (Aries, 1974, pp.55-56). In the second half of the eighteenth century, de-Christianization began to occur within Western society particularly as an expression of the Enlightenment, which encouraged the growth of science and technology and attempted to change the old morality based upon the Christian faith into one based upon secular reasoning (Kearl, 1989, p.42). Religious aspects of death rituals such as the choice of tomb, the funding of masses, etc. began to disappear, and the last will of a dying person was reduced to a secularized legal document as it is in modern times (Aries, 1974, p.64). The Enlightenment of the eighteenth century encouraged humans to think of the events of the world rationally, emphasizing 'reason', 'rationality', and 'objectivity', without any dependency, as in previous centuries, upon external authorities such as God, religion, and the church. Therefore, secular philosophies were developed which can be related to the secularization of wills described above, and had an important role in the development of medical ethics.

The political revolutions in the late eighteenth and the first half of the nineteenth century, which aimed at creating idealistic communities, led to people being interested in death, and this was reflected in their artistic activities, rituals of mourning, and the emergence of spiritualist movements. It seemed that secular individualism without a Christian connection was strengthened by the Enlightenment and the political revolutions of the eighteenth century, and made an individual aware of his private self. This idea of the unique self was considered to be significant only through the realization of different other selves, and that was why people were more concerned with the life and death of others than that of themselves at this period (Kearl, 1989, p.43) which is sometimes called the era of 'hysterical mourning' as Mark Twain's 'The California Tale' of 1893 illustrated. In this story, a man cannot accept the death of his wife even after nineteen years and continues to await her return by celebrating the anniversary of her death. Such an exaggeration of mourning tends to suggest a difficulty in the acceptance of the death of another person (Aries, 1974, pp.67-68).

The Twentieth Century - the Modern Period

The Struggle against Death After the First World War, 'mass education and mass communication, total war, the considerable differentiation and specialization of the world of work, and a near-total secularization of the everyday world' created 'a new kind of identity, a new kind of dying, and a new kind of grief' (Kearl, 1989, p.46). Individuals tended to lose intrinsic value and become just a means to an end for others and organizations (p.46). An individual's death had little influence on the society (Aries, 1981, p.560). With the dramatic pace of social changes, the complexity of social life, and different moral values, individuals became confused about how to deal with the matter of death (Kearl, 1989, p.46).

Death as a Failure In modern society, death is understood as a failure or a defeat of humans, while mass communication encourages individuals to remain eternally youthful, and this social attitude leads them to the idea that getting old (the process involving the inevitable approach of death) entails becoming imperfect and so to a feeling of guilt about it (Manning, 1984, pp.23-24). Individuals begin to deny their own mortality and their own ageing process, while they conceal the death of their relatives (Kearl, 1989, p.47).

Dread of Insignificant Extinction Death is likely to be limited largely to the elderly in contemporary society, because medicine has become able to cure many diseases, which used to be incurable in former centuries, and to prevent some of them by for example warning against cigarettes. Most people die after retiring from work or other social roles (Kearl, 1989, p.93). The need for achievement, self-esteem, and self-actualization seem much stronger in modern times than in the early Christian era because of the rise of individualism and the Enlightenment. So death without satisfying one's needs or fulfilling one's goals is shameful, and people feel mediocre through being forced to be disengaged from work or other social roles. Ironically, people normally have enough time to feel this dread of insignificant extinction in nursing homes, hospitals or hospices because medicine has succeeded in prolonging life.

A Fear of Losing Control in the Dying Process With cancer, the dying process may often not only be long but also painful and humiliating. The use of technology such as life-support machines extends not only the person's life but also the pain of his disease, and it brings life and death under the control of doctors and machines.

The Breakdown of the Nuclear Family Since the industrial revolution, children have not always been interested in taking over their parents' jobs and assuming their role in life. Hence parents have lost the role of teaching their skills and knowledge to their children, and a gap has opened up between the different generations, which has fragmented their lives together. As the young are separated from the old, the deaths of the elderly become unfamiliar to young people. Taking care of elderly parents used to be accepted as the natural responsibility of children and grandchildren, and they used to be cared for and die at home, in familiar surroundings and with dignity. With the breakdown of the nuclear family, the death of the elderly becomes hidden from their grandchildren. Children are kept away from death and are not even allowed into hospitals, and this creates a fear of death because it is unfamiliar in their daily life.

The Denial of Emotion After the Enlightenment, the West began to put on a mask in the face of death which was expressed in suffering and mourning:

> [I]n Western society there is little encouragement from an individual's social circle to talk or express feelings, and those who put on a 'public mask' and suppress their grief are rewarded and seen to be coping well. (Faulkner, 1993, p.71)

'Coping well' may mean that the person is regarded as normal, but someone who does not 'cope well' may be regarded as abnormal. In order to be considered normal, people hide their emotions and grieve in private, otherwise the society may treat them as if they were infectious (Gorer, 1964, p.31). One has to control one's emotions rationally and must not show one's weakness to others. People hide their emotions or weakness in front of their friends but go for help to 'strangers' in organizations which support the suicidal, the bereaved, the alcoholic, etc. As an adult, you are expected to deal with your emotion properly; and when you cannot do so by yourself, you should go to strange professionals, to mend 'your torn mask' and so cover your vulnerable human face by concealing your real emotion from others. You are not allowed to take your mask off in society except in front of professionals (psychologist, doctor, nurse, social worker, etc.) who are specially trained and have some 'immunity' to seeing one's 'vulnerable face' underneath the mask - no matter how ugly and distorted that face is! When you show your vulnerable face before those without 'immunity', they may run away from or ignore you, and in extreme cases go to an 'immunized' professional to talk over their 'shock' of seeing your face without the mask, and to recall also their own 'vulnerable faces', which have been forgotten for a long time.

So it is understandable that society's attitude to the emotions related to death and dying is not open but denied. In other words, 'the society has to avoid the disturbance and the overly strong and unbearable emotion caused by the ugliness of the dying and by the very presence of death in the midst of a happy life' (Aries, 1974, p.87). For example, Gorer claims that the British hide their grief in front of others and behave as if nothing had happened, and that the majority of the contemporary British do not have any appropriate idea of how to deal with death and losing their loved ones (Gorer, 1964, p.86, p.174). The subject of death becomes pornographic, being hidden in society, as sexual things were in earlier times (Gorer, 1964, p.179). But death is often ignored even in private life, and this contrasts with former responses to sexual matters where people could enjoy sex privately or get some kind of self-consolation from looking at erotic pictures in secret in order to satisfy their sexual desire, even though this was not made public. When the thought of death and the feeling of grief arise, we tend to divert them by doing something else such as working hard, watching TV, taking drugs, drinking alcohol, etc. So in modern society individuals shut the door on death and natural emotions related to death even in their private life, and in this context the taboo of death is different from the taboo of sexual issues in earlier times.

Death Rituals and Emotions We need to remember the fact that religious rituals for death still exist in the modern civilized Western world despite the de-Christianization that has occurred particularly since the Enlightenment. The meaning of religious funerals is, however, different in the modern age from that of former times, because the majority of Western people no longer seriously practice their religion in daily life. For example, Gorer discovered that less than half of the British people pray privately everyday and more than two thirds do not go to church even once a month (Gorer, 1964, p.174). He explains that there is no longer a strong fear of or faith in the Last Judgment and eternal punishment in modern Britain (p.23), and the traditional Christian rituals for the dead do not give any guidance for people in dealing with their bereavement or with someone in grief any more (p.31). On the other hand, Christian death rituals may help a dead person's family and friends psychologically to allow them to cry and show their emotions at least during the funeral (Chapter 2), and many people still believe in some idea of a life after death and hope to meet their dead relatives again (Gorer, 1964, appendix 4, pp.37-38). Faith in life after death, the resurrection, and meeting the dead again do not come however from people's serious practice of religion in their day-to-day lives but from tradition, so even if many people believe these ideas, it does not mean they have a strong faith which helps them to cope with bereavement or painful emotions in the hope of life after death. The role of Christianity is very different in the modern period from the time before the Enlightenment, when people had a real hope of resurrection, because modern Western society tends to use religious funerals as a temporary consolation and a temporary recurrence of their faith just because of tradition. But the tradition itself may work only at a surface level, just like people enjoy celebrating Christmas not necessarily thinking about its religious meaning and origin, and this does not seem to help people to deal with death and the emotions related to death.

Contemporary societies in English speaking Protestant countries deny the need for bereavement after funerals, and this tends to produce embarrassment when meeting with bereaved persons and encouragement for them to think about something else to keep them busy. From this stance, sadness and grief are not considered a natural reaction to the experience of losing loved ones but as weakness, selfishness, and bad habits (Gorer, 1964, p.178). The transition from the current religious funeral, in which people are allowed to share and express their emotions, back to secular daily life, in which people are required to hide their emotions and grief, seems to be forced to occur quickly in a very short period, as if emotions were like a machine that can be easily turned 'on' and 'off'. While the Christian tradition still continues with regard to funerals and the treatment of the dead so, for example, cremation still does not always take place in the modern Western world, this does not mean that it helps people to deal with their bereavement and to come to terms with death because the Christian tradition tends to exist only on the surface. We have described people's (particularly the British) reserved attitudes to bereavement in relation to a decline in Christian faith and rituals. Since Gorer's research was undertaken in the 1960s, some thirty years ago, we may expect that the degree of de-Christianization and prohibition on expressing emotions will have become even greater since then, as the Western world is becoming even more secularized.

Kubler-Ross' Five Psychological Stages Concerning the Dying Process
Elizabeth Kubler-Ross introduced five psychological stages in the process of dying after interviewing over two hundred dying patients (Kubler-Ross, 1969, pp.34-138). Her research took place in the 1960s, so we cannot be sure that her interpretation would be universal as an explanation of the Western attitude to death and dying at different times. But it is safe to take it as representative of the modern attitude. Let us explain the five stages here:

The first stage: denial and isolation After shock and numbness caused by the diagnosis of her incurable disease, the patient begins by denying the fact that she has got an incurable disease or she is going to die. She may sometimes go to one doctor after another for examination after examination. She is afraid to communicate with medical staff, who may tell her the reality of her coming death, and may try to pretend to herself that she is not dying. As a result, this denial leads her into a feeling of isolation. However only three of her two hundred patients, says Kubler-Ross, tried to deny their death until the end of their life.

> Most patients do not use denial so extensively. They may briefly talk about the reality of their situation, and suddenly indicate their inability to look at it realistically any longer. (Kubler-Ross, 1969, pp.36-37)

One of the reasons for denial of death is related to the fact that, as we have previously described in this section, in the modern period, death and dying have become frightening.

The second stage: anger When the patient goes beyond the denial stage, the next stage is, according to Kubler-Ross, anger, rage, envy, and resentment, and the question of 'why me?' The question 'why me?' seems to be addressed to God or any supernatural power, who is considered to be able to interfere with one's own life and death, though the questioner may not always be aware of it.

The third stage: bargaining In this stage the patient attempts to delay her inevitable death (e.g. until 'my son's wedding', 'my next birthday', etc.) by bargaining with God. She may say 'I will never ask anything more if this wish is granted'.

With regard to the second stage (the anger of 'why me?') and the third stage (bargaining), even in the secularized modern Western world, with those who do not practice any faith, we can see that religious symbols still remain in the secular Western mind in the way people face death and dying as seen in Chapter 2.

The fourth stage: depression   Depression is deeply connected with many losses which the patient has to endure, and Kubler-Ross divided the patient's depression into two sorts: reactive and preparatory depression. The reactive depression is to partial losses such as loss of body parts (breast, uterus, leg, etc.), appearance, job, and so on.   The preparatory depression is an anticipation of losses predicted in the future including body parts, appearance, and life itself.

The fifth stage: acceptance   Finally the patient will reach a stage of acceptance of his fate without depression or anger about it if he has been given some help in working through the previous four stages, in which he has been allowed to express his anger, envy, guilt, and fear.   This is not a mere hopeless resignation or giving up but like 'the final rest before the long journey' (as phrased by one patient of Kubler-Ross; Kubler-Ross, 1969, p.100), which may imply a degree of peace and contemplation.

We have described the five psychological stages of the patient in his or her dying process.   According to Kubler-Ross' analysis, throughout the five stages the patient continues to hope that she may not die (Kubler-Ross, 1969, pp.34-138).

Shneidman, also a distinguished researcher on death, argues that there is no such a thing as 'stages' which occur in this order in the dying process, and while accepting that denial, isolation, anger, bargaining, depression, and acceptance can be observed, suggests that they occur randomly not at regular intervals (Shneidman, 1986, p.7).   Manning indicates in a similar vein:

> This conceptual framework for understanding the process of dying and our established ways of dealing with death is not intended to be taken rigidly; a very common misconception about these 'stages' is that they always occur uniformly and in sequence.   (Manning, 1984, pp.28-29)

However, it is almost impossible to exclude the nuance that a 'certain order' exists in the psychological process of dying from using an expression like 'stages'.   If they do not always occur in the order of the five stages, nor all patients always experience all stages, then we have to ask why Kubler-Ross uses the term 'stages', which itself implies 'an order' and 'uniformity'.

Nevertheless, Kubler-Ross's investigation and analysis do reveal the modern Western attitude to death and dying. Until reaching the fifth stage of acceptance (if one does ever reach it), the image of death seems to be rather negative as the first four stages involve something to deny, resent, postpone, and be depressed about. These attitudes are deeply related to the fear of death described earlier in this section; in other words, the fear intensifies these reactions. Moreover, the idea of 'stages' in the dying process is more feasible in the modern period, when the dying process becomes longer (and often painful), and the birth of such an idea of 'stages' is itself an expression of the modern nature of the dying process.

The Western Hospice Movement and Attitude to Death and Dying

In the first section of this chapter, we explored how the Western attitude to death and dying has changed throughout history. Now let us consider the historical connection between the hospice movement and the changing Western attitude to death and dying, in order to understand the underlying notion of the hospice movement in terms of attitudes to death and dying.

The Medieval Ages

From the twelfth century, with the beginning of the discovery of an individual self, people began to be more aware of their own death and responsibilities for their deeds and to take more notice of the Christian idea of the Last Judgment. This led them to repent of their sins and earnestly desire to gain salvation. So, to some extent, the spread of hospices in this period was linked with people's actions based upon the fear of death, and it is interesting to notice that the time when the fear of death began coincided with the period when hospices began to flourish. Overcoming the fear of death and the Last Judgment was achieved by making a pilgrimage to attain salvation, which allowed one to go to heaven and be resurrected.

The Eighteenth and Nineteenth Centuries

A dramatic change occurred in both the attitude to death and the hospice at the time of the Enlightenment. A change of hospitals from 'refuges' into places for the care of the sick with clinical functions was seen in this period. With the emergence of medical science, hospitals made every effort to cure patients rather than simply care for them, so the idea of the care-centred hospice of previous ages was no longer of interest. Secularisation of day-to-day life with the emphasis on reasoning and rationality led to de-Christianization. So the way of overcoming the fear of death was to be attained not by the hope of going to heaven or faith in resurrection, but by 'conquering death' using scientific medical technologies to cure diseases or prolong the life of the dying as much as possible. This tendency of fighting against death, to the end, made the dying process more frightening by encouraging painful aggressive treatments and the dehumanization of patients. From this time, the West began to deal with death mainly by denying it, and this changed the notion of death from a natural event into a shameful and dreadful one.

The problems, to which the modern hospice movement has lately reacted, began to be created at this time, and the care-centred hospice of the medieval ages maintained by nursing religious orders throughout this difficult period has played an extremely important role in the modern hospice movement.

The Modern Period (the Twentieth Century)

Modern society denies and avoids talking about not only death but also the ageing process and emotional issues related to it. Death and the dying processes are even more frightening in the increasingly secularized world than in the previous century. One person's death has little influence on a society with no religious faith in day-to-day life except the practising of religious rituals at a superficial level and only on special occasions such as funerals and weddings; with the idea of a person's life being merely for achievement and self-esteem; with no intrinsic value of the individual; and with the open expression of emotions seen as weakness, embarrassing, and abnormal. In these social circumstances, the modern hospice movement developed as a strong reaction against the modern cure-centred hospital and its associated attitude to death and dying.

Modern hospices' attitudes to death and cancer patients have a remarkable correlation to the Western attitude to death in the early Christian era, which we have already considered in the first section. In the early Christian period until the twelfth century, death was understood to be predictable: individuals could prepare for death; there was faith and hope in the resurrection; no strong awareness of the Last Judgment; and death was an act that involved the community. Modern hospices seem to be interested particularly in cancer patients, and 'the predictability of death' in the early Christian period corresponds to that of cancer patients today, whose death is more likely to be predicted than that from any other disease. 'Preparation for death' is also important in the modern hospice, which provides spiritual as well as psychological care and lets patients gain peace of mind by 'forgiveness of sins' as we have explored in the section on the pilgrim-cancer patient metaphor (Chapter 2). 'Faith and hope in heaven and the resurrection', may not exist in the modern hospice in the same way as in early Christian times unless patients are seriously-practising Christians, but the modern hospice may still try to help patients to achieve 'heaven and resurrection' in a metaphorical sense. The modern hospice may help patients discover 'heaven within themselves' in the process of dying by giving every possible treatment in preventing and controlling their pains and by helping them to reach a peaceful state of mind. As St Luke's Gospel says ' ... the kingdom of God is within you' (Luke 17: 21).

Also, patients may 'be resurrected' by becoming 'new persons' after spiritual development through reflection on their lives and forgiveness of themselves as well as others. As to there being 'no strong awareness of the Last Judgement', modern patients may not have a strong idea or fear of their Last Judgment in the same way as in the early Christian period, though the reason for this is very different in each case. For the former, it is because of loss of Christian faith; for the latter because there was no strong awareness of an individual self. Finally, 'death as an event involving the community' may be possible in the modern hospice to a certain degree. The patient's family plays an important role in caring for and dealing with the patient, and strong emotions such as grief and bereavement are allowed to be expressed within hospice care, so the patient's family and caring staff can share the event of death and the dying process within the community called a 'hospice'.

Another interesting point is that both medieval and modern 'pilgrimages' began, to some extent, out of fear of death and dying. The twelfth century was the time when 'hospices' as shelters for pilgrims began to flourish and also when people increased their awareness of the individual self, individual responsibility for good and bad deeds in life, and the Last Judgment, which made them conscious of fear of death and led them to take pilgrimages. As pilgrimages increased, the demand for hospices must have become high, so that tired pilgrims on the road to shrines could be cared for. In regard to modern hospices, they were established as a reaction against the modern hospital and its way of treating dying cancer patients. They have gained great support from the general public, and this may be related to their fear of a painful and shameful death in hospital. As medieval people took their pilgrimage partly because of fear of death and overcame the fear through their Christian faith in salvation, the notion of modern hospices may try to relate fear of death and 'pilgrimage' once again. So, fear of death seems to be one of the important factors both for the medieval and the modern hospice.

Modern hospice patients and people in early Christian times share certain similar circumstances, and the modern hospice attempts, in its philosophy, either consciously or unconsciously, to revive the old attitudes to death and dying for contemporary Western society. This attempt has, however, a limitation because there is a stronger fear and individual awareness of death in the modern period, compared with the early Christian period.

However, we should not forget the paradoxical nature of the modern Western hospice movement in its attitude to death, dying, and emotions. While the modern hospice has developed as a strong reaction against the modern attitude to death, the care of the dying, and emotions related to them, it is ironic to find these same attitudes reflected in the nature of the hospice movement. This is because, as we have elucidated in the pilgrim-cancer patient metaphor, the hospice tends to isolate the matter of death, dying, and bereavement from the world outside hospice care and so may prevent a more fundamental examination. People have to depend upon hospice care when they or their loved ones get cancer or are bereaved, because there is nowhere for them to go otherwise. Society tends to support the hospice movement financially but this does not itself change the society's attitude to death, dying and their associated emotions. So the philosophy of hospice care may not have a strong influence on the public mind, as was explained in the analogy of the 'greenhouse' and 'strawberries' (Chapter 2). The presence of the hospice itself tends to demonstrate evidence of society's denial of death and emotions, and the reason why cancer patients are forced to be 'pilgrims' in the modern period has to be considered with the modern attitude to death and emotions in mind, as we discussed in the preceding chapter. We see, therefore, that the modern hospice movement is against the modern attitude to death, dying, and their associated emotions but at the same time, in a sense, reinforces them.

Finally, we indicated in chapter 2 that religious connotations in the hospice philosophy as seen in the pilgrim-cancer patient metaphor do not always exist in a strong sense but can remain as a symbol even if some modern hospices are now more secularized. The notion of the patient's anger of 'why me?' and bargaining as introduced in Kubler-Ross's five psychological stages on the dying process are a good example of symbols which have religious roots but have become secularized in the modern Western mind. These symbols, even if the patient may not be aware of their religious meaning, easily fit the idea of 'sin' and 'penitence' in the pilgrim-cancer patient metaphor.

6 The Japanese Attitude to Death and Dying

Introduction

In this chapter, we will analyze the relationship between the Japanese way of delivering hospice care and the Japanese attitude to death and dying: in the first section, we will look at how people have perceived the matter of death and dying in history from classic to modern times; and in the second section we will consider the relationship between the hospice and the attitude to death and dying.

History of the Japanese Attitude to Death and Dying

Until the Period of Nara (to 710 AD)

Before the arrival of Buddhism in the sixth century, there was a traditional religion known as 'Shinto' in Japan, whose faith rests on the idea that God founded this world by descending from heaven and establishing a state of affairs where Heaven and Earth became separated, and trees and herbs spoke. According to this belief, there are many deities in Japan, and the supreme deity is the sun-goddess (Anesaki, 1930, pp.19-20). In Shinto there is belief in the dead person's resurrection, as represented in the custom of 'Mogari', which is found in *Gishi-wajin-den*, a Chinese history book written in the third century. During the period of 'Mogari', a family drank and danced gathering together for more than ten days, after which the dead body was finally buried. Finishing the burial, they entered into the water to purify their bodies (Inoue, 1986, p.177). There are two paradoxical attitudes to the dead in this custom, first that people feared the dead while they expected their resurrection; and second that death was understood as a phenomenon in which a person's spirit left his body temporarily and went to 'somewhere' but would come back as long as the body remained (Enmaru, 1978, p.137).

A lot of earthenware has been excavated from tombs dating from the sixth century onwards. People must have thought that the life-style in the next world would not be very different from this world, because earthenware used in their daily life was buried with the dead body in the tomb (Enmaru, 1978, p.142). The name of the next world was 'Yomi-no-kuni' as reported in a Japanese classic *Koji-ki* completed in the early eighth century, where Izanagi visited his wife Izanami in 'Yomi-no-kuni'. No longer was the world after death just 'somewhere' as it had been thought of in former centuries, but a place near this world like 'Yomi-no-kuni' which could be visited easily. In Shinto it is believed that both the good and the bad go to 'Yomi-no-kuni' after death, so there is no idea similar to the Last Judgment as found in Christianity.

The cremation of dead bodies began after Buddhism was made public in 538 AD. The first cremation on record in Japan was that of a priest named Dosho in 700 AD. There are two main streams in Buddhism: (i) Jodomon - as a result of good deeds in this life, one can be born in 'Saiho-jodo' (the Pure Land) after death; (ii) Shodomon - one can reach the state of mind rising above life and death by 'satori' (spiritual enlightenment) in this world, but not in the next world. Both Jodomon and Shodomon emphasize the spiritual aspect of life rather than the existence of the body, in order to be born in the Pure Land after death in the former, or transcend death itself in the latter (Kino, 1986, pp.130-40). But Buddhism was not popularized until the twelfth century, when it no longer emphasized its philosophical purity but was simplified to suit the ordinary Japanese perspective on the world (Becker, 1994). So the introduction of Buddhism to Japan did not have a strong influence on ordinary people's attitudes to death and dying during the period of Nara, which was more Shintoistic.

The Periods of Heian and Kamakura (C9th-C14th)

The dead body was thought to have some spiritual power at the beginning of the ninth century, as we find in *Nihon-reii-ki* written in the early ninth century collection of legendary myths in Japan. One of the stories tells that a dead body of the victim of murder discerned a person who was his assailant (Watanabe, 1988, p.105), and it is interesting that a dead body was seen as remaining a person who had some social role like that of discerning an assailant.

While faith by easy and simple methods was demanded, Kuya taught a mere invocation of the name of Buddha and its power for salvation (Saunders, 1964, p.137). Genshin, a founder of the Jodo sect of Buddhism took this idea and taught that the repetition of the nembutsu (invocation of the name of Amida, a Buddha - from the Sanskrit: Amitabha) helped humans to be saved and reborn in the Western Paradise (or the Pure Land). He wrote a book entitled *Ojoyoshu, A Collection of Essentials Concerning Rebirth in the Western Paradise* (i.e., Amida's Western Paradise), which vividly described the paradise. During the political catastrophe of the twelfth century, Honen (1133-1212), inspired by Genshin's work *Ojoyoshu*, established the Pure Land sect (the Jodo sect) ordering and teaching the Amidist precept (Saunders, 1964, pp.191-92).

A real popularization of Buddhism began from this time, and the Pure Land sect has been one of the most popular Buddhist sects amongst lay Japanese since then until modern times. The important thing here is that the idea emphasized by persons like Genshin and Honen tends to be based upon a belief in the inability of men to help themselves in reaching salvation and also their need for practical and easier methods for salvation such as mere repetitions of the name of Amida. Although there is an idea of hell in the Jodo sect of Buddhism, the image of hell and the Last Judgment became weakened because of the belief that every sort of deadly sinner, will be saved by repeating the name of Amida.

Sagara Ryo interprets the Japanese feeling of death as something sad ('kanashii') rather than frightening, through analysing two famous Japanese classics, *Genji-monogatari* completed in the early eleventh century and *Heike-monogatari* written at the end of twelfth century. *Genji-monogatari* is a novel telling of a handsome hero who is a son of the Emperor. Despite his noble birth and being loved by many women, he is not happy but lonely. When his loved one named Murasakinoue passes away, he says in deep grief that he feels relieved recognizing what his life is like and how he himself is situated. He finally understands that life is sad and transient. This conclusion is reflected in his attitude to death. Death is sad in the same way as life is. Appreciating this truth, he can feel relieved, because he becomes able to accept the sadness of human life as it is, though this does not mean that he no longer sorrows. He decides to become a priest giving up every attachment to this world (Sagara, 1984, pp.39-46).

Heike-monogatari is based upon a true story of the defeat of Heike (the Hei or Taira clan). Sagara thinks that the author depicted 'Aware' (sadness or compassion) of the Taira clan's warriors in an inescapable destiny under the feudal system, where committing suicide because of the defeat of their clan meant loyalty to their master or clan, but surviving was an act of treachery. In their solidarity, death seemed to be considered as a destiny which an individual could not control by himself alone, and the notion of 'Aware' (sadness or compassion) arises from the fact that people had to face this unavoidable destiny of their community (Sagara, 1984, pp.74-76).

While they were searching for honour, they had to give up their lives, being good losers, and rush into death actively and manfully when they faced their defeat. This enlightenment (kakugo) of warriors is different from that (satori) of Buddhism, which transcends life and death, and does not feel sad about death (Sagara, 1984, p.17, p.112). In the warrior's 'kakugo', death was a sad destiny, but he accepted the destiny and bore the sadness so that he could die with dignity and honour (pp.112-14). Most ordinary people were not considered to reach such a state of mind in the Buddhist or the warrior's way, and so the easier method of salvation of the Jodo sect in Buddhism became popular throughout the centuries. Because the majority of people could not overcome the sadness of death, they asked Amida to save them by their simple faith. So we find that ordinary people passively gave up their destiny and depended upon the mercy of Amida to overcome their sadness, accepting their inability to save themselves from death or from hell, and to overcome sadness.

A ceremony of warriors' suicide 'Seppuku' (or 'Harakiri'), which began in 1170 (by Minamoto-no-Tametomo) and 1180 (by Minamoto-no-Yorimasa) expresses the warrior's attitude to death. 'Seppuku' (cutting one's abdomen by using a short sword) was carried out to avoid being killed by enemies and living in shame, and to die with dignity and peace. As soon as 'Seppuku' was completed a companion 'kaishakunin' standing behind the suicidal person cut his head off to stop the pain caused by his 'Seppuku'. Therefore the warrior was supposed to die a peaceful and honourable death without dramatic physical pain (Becker, 1989, pp.156-57), though the sadness of his death is to be found in his farewell poem.

From the first half of the thirteenth century, Dogen began Zen training. Rejecting an understanding of the world through reasoning and logic, the Zennist attempts to transcend the usual way of thinking. He believes that there is an ego, but that it is cosmic not individual, and is to be realized in every soul at the same time, being the ultimate reality transcending all individual differences. In other words, people essentially originated in a sole existence called the SOUL or MIND. Once an individual identifies himself with the whole cosmos, he is no longer troubled by incidents such as death. Zen was used for military men so that they did not have to fear death but could control their minds with firmness so that they were led to a spiritually high level (Anesaki, 1930, pp.206-10). Probably very few people reached this spiritual state though, but felt sad about their destiny in the same way as already described through *Heike-monogatari*.

The Periods of Namboku-cho and Muromachi (C14th-C17th)

Anesaki describes clearly the political conditions in this period:

> [A]s a result of the weakness of the dictator (Shogun) selfish motives and relentless strife were rampant. The Emperor was treated as a puppet by the Shogun, the latter in turn by his Commissioners (Shikken), who were again abused by their majordomos (Shitsuji), and lower retainers ... The Zen ideal of 'beyond good and bad' was abused to an extreme of 'nothing good or bad'. (Anesaki, 1930, pp.215-16)

In this unstable political situation there was pessimism about one's position or wealth, which was not secure. *Taihei-ki*, completed before 1371, narrates humans' desires and struggles in the rise and fall of their fortune at that time. The book shows the meaninglessness of the Buddhist idea for politics, in explaining that this world is in desperate darkness, where we are dealt with by fate, except for just a short period of peace. Although Buddhism makes much of transcending fate, *Taihei-ki* faces the reality in which people are subject to fate. The attitude towards death in *Taihei-ki* is contrasted with that of *Heike-monogatari*. In *Taihei-ki*, people do not follow their destiny of defeat but show resistance in this world, while those in *Heike-monogatari* accept their fate with sadness. Resistance against fate and death in the former tends to be manifest in the cruel manner of their death, which we do not find in the latter. For example, in the description of Nitta Yoshisada's death, he tries to hide his head after cutting it off by himself. This gruesome scene typifies this dark age, where death and dying appear to be cruel (Sagara, 1984, pp.79-109).

The Period of Edo (C17th-C19th)

There are two pieces of literature which teach 'Mugen-kan' (regarding life merely as a dream or phantasm): (i) *Mikawa-monogatari* (1622); (ii) *Hagakure* (completed before 1716). The author of the former teaches that this world is a temporary house (the evanescent world), so there is no meaning in pursuing prosperity here. The latter says that a person is like a marionette worked by someone and human life is not stable. Both writers believe that the only meaningful thing to do in this world is to live for their lord and treasure the master-man relationship giving up any sort of attachment to the world. It seems that the authors attempt to revive the spirit of the warrior as it existed before the seventeenth century (Sagara, 1984, pp.121-51).

After the middle of the Edo Period, *Ojo-den* (a book about an ideal death) was translated into Japanese, having been written in Chinese before but only being read by the educated such as Court people and warriors. In Japan though, *Ojo-den* became popular amongst the general public, and Ryuen edited sixteen volumes of *Ojo-den* titled *Kinsei ojo-den* (the modern age *Ojo-den*). According to *Kinsei Ojo-den*, there were many people who died peacefully and happily believing in Buddha and saying 'Nembutsu' (the name of Buddha). Around the death bed, a good scent drifted in the air, and beautiful music was heard from somewhere, which was called 'Zuisou' (Watanabe, 1988, pp.85-86). This may be interpreted, either through the revival of the warrior's spirit or 'Zuisou', as the people of the Edo Period seeking after the ideal way of death in the midst of a peaceful social atmosphere.

However death was still sad. Motoori Norinaga (1730-1801), a Japanese classical scholar, saw that death was to be absorbed in the world of the Gods and going to 'Yomi-no-kuni' was inevitable as 'Shinto' taught. Motoori said that people could be at peace by accepting death as a destiny that was unavoidable, and could only mourn because it was natural to feel so. Since whatever happens in this world comes from the will of the gods, through feeling sad over what is naturally saddening, we can be harmonized with the gods and get relief (Sagara, 1984, pp.20-28).

The Period of Meiji and After (C19th-C20th)

By opening itself to foreign trade and diplomatic relations since the Meiji Restoration, and particularly after the Second World War, Japan has imported Western philosophy and a Westernized education system. The high economic growth in the twentieth century (particularly since the 1960s) caused the structure of Japanese society to become highly urbanized and industrialized. In these circumstances, many people do not take up their parents' occupations, and this breaks traditional connections between the old and young generations. Through the increasing emergence of the nuclear family, children become unable to see their grandparents' death. Meanwhile, the dramatic development of medical technology enables the Japanese to prolong their lives at the same time as death and dying are becoming far removed from their daily lives. Death and dying tend not to be observed except through TV or films.

However, the elderly and cancer patients in Japan have particular problems in facing painful and ugly deaths. In contemporary Japanese society, after developing an incurable disease, people usually live for a long period in a hospital controlled by doctors. During this period, the patient is made to feel ashamed of troubling his attendant and showing his pitiable figure in incontinence pads and on life-support equipment, since Japanese culture always requires one to care about how others feel about him or her. There is a shrine called 'Pokkuri Jinja' where the elderly go to pray for their speedy death (Watanabe, 1988, pp.16-17). Most of the doctors and nurses who have not received any special education about death and dying often concentrate only on physical care, trying to ignore the patient's loneliness, anxiety, sadness, and fear of death as well as their own fear (Chapter 3). Besides these psychological pains, patients often have the physical pain of diseases such as cancer. Although a peaceful state of mind in relation to death and dying was respected in former centuries, dying patients in modern hospitals may not be able to be at peace because their pain is unnaturally prolonged as a result of the extreme activities of doctors attempting to postpone death. Moreover, Japanese people usually die after retirement from work at about 55-60 years of age. As already mentioned, the emergence of nuclear families destroys a strong link between the young and the old, so the social role of old people within the family is disappearing. Thus, in the modern era, people tend to die in old age not needed by society.

Even the Showa Emperor spent 111 days in the hospital of the Imperial Household Agency, not told the truth that he had got incurable cancer but given every possible treatment for life-prolongation. TV, radio, and newspapers reported his condition every day, with such expressions as 'He is stable at this moment' but never mentioned the name of his disease. During his stay in hospital there were two interesting reactions found amongst Japanese citizens. One was that rich Japanese patients in many hospitals asked doctors to give them similar treatment to the Emperor; another was that many Japanese, shocked to hear of the extreme prolongation of the Emperor's life pleaded not to be given such care at their death, and became members of the Japan Society for Dying with Dignity. The rich patients might not have wanted the same treatment as the Emperor, if they had known that it prolonged his severe pain for

111 days (Oki, 1991, pp.3-4).

In facing the reality of dying without dignity, the old, the dying, and their families have begun to talk about death and dying frankly. The mass media have taken their voice seriously and let the public know the fact that there are many people like the Emperor who are dying with long-term suffering and without dignity, controlled almost entirely by doctors, and not told the nature of their disease (Watanabe, 1988, pp.13-14). Given this information, the general public has paid attention to thinking about and discussing matters of death and dying, which have been neglected by recent generations. Therefore it is understandable that the topic of death and dying has been pre-eminent amongst both the intelligentsia and the general public in Japanese society for some ten years. Responding to this, the mass media have made various programmes about death and dying: euthanasia; brain death; suicide; near-death experience; life after death; how to organize a funeral; the land problem concerning graves; psychic phenomena and shows; new religions, etc. Some treat death and dying seriously, but others, just out of curiosity, for example, introducing different methods of suicide with a phrase such as 'Have them handy so you can do it whenever you want!' (SPA!, 1991, p.29, translated by myself).

The treatment of the dying has changed in the modern period, because of the high-technology of medical science, which has made the nature of the dying process more frightening and painful as we have seen. However, the Japanese attitude to death and dying has remained traditional in other respects, since Japanese people still tend to react to someone's death and dying in traditional ways. One of the big factors is that Japan is not an individualistic society, so that death and dying cannot be readily privatized. This is despite the fact that Japan has been awakened to the idea of individualism and the search has begun for personal goals in life related to economic development through the influence of Western education and philosophy. Japanese individualism is only just beginning and may possibly be different in its meaning from Western individualism. While a discontinuity between the young and old has begun to appear and the number of nuclear families has begun to increase, Japanese people are still not independent of the family or group, as Becker explains:

A person who made independent decisions would be the worst kind of person in Japanese society. Rather the entire culture and the language itself assure that Japanese people will always consider other people in making their decisions. This education begins in their youngest years and continues throughout life. (Becker, 1992, p.249; translated by Becker)

If Becker's point of view is accurate, in this social climate, death may be still not an event of the individual but of the family or group even in the modern period. Watsuji Tetsuro mentions that the Japanese word for 'person' (Ningen: Nin means 'person' and Gen, 'relationship') does not imply an individual but a relationship with others. The concept of 'Ningen' appears in the Japanese attitude to a dead person's body. The dead person is not a thing but still a person until his body is cremated and buried (Becker, 1992, pp.253-54). We might say that even a dead body plays an important role in maintaining connections amongst members of the family or group.

The existence of a dead person's body reminds the family of his social role and encourages its members to recover its strong connections and, therefore, in this sense, a dead body is not different from a living person in the Japanese mind. For example, after the Japan Airlines aeroplane crash in 1985, teams of people tried to find the victims' bodies taking a few weeks to do so. The families who had not yet had their loved ones' bodies back, eventually went to the actual spot of the tragedy (though it was a high mountain) and prayed for the repose of the souls of the dead (Becker, 1992, p.254; Sasaki, 1986, p.152). Another example is that even fifty years after the second world war, Japanese families have not given up looking for the bones of their relatives and loved ones, who were killed during the war, in China and the Philippines (Becker, 1992, p.254). The origins of this attachment to the body are not found in Buddhism but in Shinto, as seen earlier, but the Japanese tend to treasure the dead body whether they are Buddhist or Shintoist, and this applies even though the majority of modern Japanese do not practise either religion.

Not only respect for but also the fear of a dead body still remains, to a certain degree, in modern Japanese society. For example, in the hospital 'Futsurei' (Purification ceremony) is often conducted at the entrance of the mortuary when a dead body is carried there, for the purpose of avoiding any disturbance of the spirits of other dead bodies which used to be in the room before a new dead body's arrival (Sasaki, 1986, pp.153-54). Hands are also purified by salt after touching a dead body. Such respect for and fear of a dead body remind us of the custom of 'Mogari' in the third century.

Another important aspect to consider with regard to the traditional attitude to death and dying, which has remained in the modern period, is that many ordinary people give up fighting against their fate in the face of the reality that they will die not knowing the nature of their disease but feeling their bodies becoming weaker day by day (Kashiwagi, 1991a, p.85). This 'giving up' or 'resignation' is shared with the Japanese from earlier times, as already described. In accepting the fate brought by Nature or some supernatural power of the universe, the Japanese in the modern period may die in sadness.

The question to be raised here is about how we can understand the relationship between the Japanese attitude to death and a dead body; in other words, why the Japanese have a strong attachment to the dead bodies of their loved ones despite their having less attachment to their own life, in which they accept death as a fate to be accepted. We may find the answer in the distinction between their attitude to their own death and to others' deaths. As we have already explored, the Japanese consider their own death as something sad and an unavoidable fate so they try to accept it as a part of Nature, but perhaps they cannot accept others' deaths as easily as they can their own death. Japanese people need time to accept someone's death, and their attachment to the person's dead body may be an expression of this. Because of less self-awareness, the Japanese have a strong identification of their selves and lives with the group or family to which they belong, and the identification might be an important basis for their psychological and social security. To lose a member of their group may disturb its security so it has to re-establish the balance of human relationships and strengthen the bonds after the person's death.

Conversely, they may be able to accept their own death more easily, because the idea of extinction of an individual self does not seem to be strong in the group's nature and this prevents an individual from experiencing fear of his own death in a very private way, and also because the existential value of a dead person merged into his group or family continues to remain even after the person's death. On the living people's part, because of the fact that a dead person's existence still has an important value and meaning in their group, his death may violate their psychological or social security and may make them find it difficult or take them a long time to accept his or her death. On the other hand, for a dying person's part, because of his strong affiliation with the group or the family and his lack of self-awareness, he may not really be aware of death as a matter affecting himself as an individual and this could reduce his fear of death.

The difficulty in accepting others' death may be also shown in the fact that the barrier between life and death is not very substantial in the Japanese mind as we found in the world of death called 'Yominokuni', which is near to this world so that the dead can come and go easily. Because accepting others' death is difficult, the Japanese might want to create the idea of a world after death which is near to this world.

Concerning the unclear line between life and death, the traditional attitude still surviving in contemporary Japanese society is also to be understood in the attitude to suicide. The Japanese have no strict prohibition against suicide and the rate of suicide in Japan is higher than in the West. Kawai, a psychoanalyst, points out that the line between life and death is readily penetrable in the Japanese mind, and he gives a description from a neurotic who attempted suicide: 'To commit suicide is not such a big decision to make ... it is like going to another room by opening the paper screen sliding door (shoji) in order to escape from the room I am in now, in which the air is not fresh and I feel choked up' (Kawai, 1991, p.249, my translation). There must be many reasons for the Japanese people's relatively tolerant public attitude to suicide in the current competitive and busy society. However, the tendency to see no clear distinction between life and death in the Japanese mind must be an important background factor.

This historical analysis of the Japanese attitude to death and dying has shown that there are some important underlying attitudes which have remained throughout history. The first derives from the non-individualistic nature of the society, as shown in the Jodo sect of Buddhism which believes that everyone can go to the Pure Land if they repeat the name of Amida, or in the idea of 'Yomi-no-kuni' in the Shinto tradition, in which both the good and the bad go there after death. Therefore the processes of death and dying have been shared in the community and the lack of strong self-awareness is reflected in the Japanese people's attachment to the dead body and difficulty in accepting others' death. The second is the idea that one's death is sad and is to be accepted as a matter of fate, and in which life can never be permanent but is part of a natural cycle of the universe, and this can be a background of sadness and resignation. It may be too extreme to say that there is no fear of death but only sadness and a resignation to death in the Japanese mind, as there is an example of warriors in *Taihei-ki* in the thirteenth century, who had a strong attachment to life. However, a 'sad death' and 'resignation' are some of the most crucial features of the Japanese attitude to death and dying. The third is that the world of death is often near to this world, as we have seen in the example of the suicidal person in modern times and 'Yomi-no-kuni' in the Shinto tradition since the third century. This leads us to an unclear distinction between life and death in the Japanese mind. We will discuss some of these characteristics of the Japanese attitude to death and dying in the next section of this chapter together with the hospice movement and also in a later chapter in a comparison with the West.

The Japanese Hospice Movement and Attitude to Death and Dying

A Group Responsibility for the Matter of Death and Dying

Through the historical analysis of the Japanese attitude to death and dying in the preceding section of this chapter, we understood that the matter of death and dying has never been privatized in Japanese society but has always been an event involving a group or community, to which a dying or dead person belongs. This tendency is reflected also in the way hospice care has been arranged in Japan, in which an individual cancer patient does not die his or her own death but a surrounding circle of people decide the best for him or her, and in which normally it is the patient's family who often desire and ask for hospice care for the patient, rather than the patient himself (Chapter 3). The patient, even in a hospice ward, is often not told the fact that he or she has got an incurable cancer (Chapter 3). Individual responsibility for the disease as well as death and dying is prevented by this lack of disclosure, and others make a decision in regard to the matter of life and death on behalf of the patient. With this state of affairs, even in hospice care, it is difficult for the patient him/herself to take an initiative in the process of dying. Moreover, Japanese people, as we have analyzed, have difficulty in accepting their loved ones' death, so it is hard to popularize hospice care as 'a place (a ward) for the dying', in which the family has to (if not patients themselves) accept that patients are going to die in the near future.

The Hospice as the Dirtiest Place

As already discussed (Chapter 3), the National Institute for Cancer Research wipes all books returned by patients with alcohol before others borrow them. Cancer is not contagious, so the purpose of wiping the books has nothing to do with a hygienic concern but more to do with the image of cancer as involving 'dirt' or 'impurity' in the Japanese mind, because there is a strong idea that all sorts of diseases are associated with 'dirt' and 'impurity' and come from outside the homes or the body.

Japanese hospice care has tended to be developed inside hospitals, which are understood as dirty places, so hospice wards full of dying patients come to be regarded as even dirtier or impurer places because not only the 'dirt' of disease but also that of death are considered to be there. Mothers may say to their children in the hospital: 'Don't go in that direction ... it is a hospice ward, where there are people dying of cancer. You could get cancer! It is a very dirty place!' In fact, the Japanese word for 'hospital' is 'byo-in' in which 'byo' means illness or disease and 'in' 'the wall around a house, made of the soil or the house itself' (*Dictionary of the Chinese Character*). The original meaning of the word 'byo-in' conveys the idea of separating the disease within a house surrounded by a wall. So a special unit for dying cancer patients called a 'hospice' inside the house for the diseased separated by a wall from the outside does not conjure up a good image for Japanese people.

'Sad Death' and Hospice Care

We have explored in Chapter 3 how the Japanese tend to be resigned (akirameru) to disease and death as fate, because of their understanding of them as a part of the supernatural universe. At the same time, however, apart from the Nambokucho and Muromachi periods (C14th-C17th), it seems that to the Japanese mentality death has been something sad, and that Japanese people have not just resigned themselves or given up their life to fate but have done so with sadness. It is wrong to say that there is no fear of death for the Japanese, but 'sadness' and 'resignation' express some important dimensions of the Japanese attitude to death and dying. It is important here to think about why death is sad for them or what they are sad about. We cannot control our destiny because of impermanence and frailty, but will eventually die and be absorbed in a cycle of Nature, no matter how much we struggle. So, what Japanese people are sad about in relation to death is the impermanent and frail nature of all beings and events in the universe.

Sadness is often linked with the object of compassion; for example, you may be feeling compassion for your friend if she dies of cancer or for yourself because you lose her. But this is different from anger or fear, since 'sadness' tends to imply the fact that you accept the situation as the thing you cannot control, while anger and fear have the connotation of fighting against or controlling it because you are angry or fearful. In fear, you may sometimes want to run away from the object, and that means you do not accept it but still fight against it in a rather cowardly way. Sadness may not imply changing the situation or controlling events that happen to individuals, but in itself shows a kind of passive acceptance of the situation and events, whether individuals are happy with them or not. There may not be any anger or fear but just compassion for those including oneself involved in the situation and events. When we say 'death is sad', therefore, whether we like it or not, we accept it as something inevitable and feel compassion for ourselves, our vulnerability and frailty in our destiny. It may be possible for one to fear something which makes him sad, but once he consciously feels the fear he tries to prevent or fight against it. But if the Japanese are likely to have passively given themselves up to the fate of their own death with sadness, this must be distinguished from the fear of sadness. As we have already described, the Japanese have had a longer history of accepting the destiny of death than of fighting against it with a strong attachment to life (as in *Taihei-ki* in the thirteenth century). That is why it is thought that a 'sad death', rather than a 'frightening death', is one of the most crucial features of the Japanese attitude to death, though the modern Japanese may be afraid of the dying process becoming frightening and painful with the high technology of medical science, which has led too much to an over-institutionalized way of treating patients.

We are not sure, however, that the Japanese idea of a 'sad death' can coexist with the hospice philosophy and its Christian background imported from the West. When physical symptoms are appropriately controlled in the development of palliative medicine and aggressive treatments are stopped in hospice care, fear of the dying process will be reduced for terminal cancer patients, and they may die a 'sad death'; in other words, feeling compassion not only for themselves in the fate of death but also for all beings in this world, who are weak and will have to die sooner or later, as they will. To die a 'sad death' may mean to die as a part of Nature and to resign human potentiality with full compassion for all frail sentient beings in the world, and this may bring great peace to the dying process of an individual. This attitude is, however, a passive attitude to what will happen in the future, and different from accepting pain and disease or death actively as a 'cross' and to walk following Christ as the Christian background of hospice philosophy may stress. The Christian background of the hospice philosophy may not be able to incorporate the idea that 'death is sad' as we will examine more in the next chapter on a comparison between the West and Japan.

7 Death and Dying and the Japanese Hospice Movement

Introduction

In Chapter 4, we described similarities and differences between the Western and the Japanese hospice movement in general, limiting the range of our discussion to the issues considered in Chapters 2 and 3. Now, we will have to make a comparison between them from the aspect of the historical and cultural interpretation of death and dying, in order to clarify some problems in bringing the idea of the Western hospice movement to Japan. So the main aim of this Chapter is firstly to make a comparison between the Western and the Japanese attitude to death and dying, and secondly to elucidate how similarities and differences between the two are related to the hospice movement in Japan.

A Comparison of the Attitude to Death and Dying

Similarities

The Way in Which People Die in the Modern Era and Its Background It may be accurate to say that there are several common aspects in terms of death and dying in modern civilized countries, whether in the West or Japan. As society became urbanized, individuals began to search for their own goals in life rather than taking over their parents' jobs. This created a gap between the young and the old generations, as is shown in the increase of the nuclear family. Children have become unable to see their grandparents' death and dying. Death is, thus, becoming unfamiliar to individuals apart from fiction on TV or films. The development of medical science has succeeded in prolonging a person's life and curing diseases through increasing knowledge and technology. So it has become possible for many people to live much longer than in past centuries, and the majority of people die after retiring from their work and giving up other social roles. The discontinuity between the young and the old may make the old's life experiences and wisdom of life 'unnecessary', and make them through being disengaged from all social roles appear 'useless'. Becoming 'useless' and 'unnecessary', the elderly may face a rather painful and shameful dying process in hospital, by being connected up with a lot of tubes and machines, and being given aggressive treatments. Therefore, people today are often scared of the dying process, in which they lose independence and become very much under the control of medical professionals. The description so far is shared by both the West and Japan in the modern era.

Remaining Religious Traditions   The Enlightenment in the eighteenth century represents the beginning of de-Christianization in the West. In modern times, the majority of the Western population do not go to church or seriously believe in God even if they go to church. The place for God in their life seems to have been replaced by science, which offers a cause-effect relationship for events in the world, and a logical as well as a rational way of dealing with problems. It is as if humans might have already sat on 'the throne of God'. Despite such secularization of the Western mind, many people organize funerals in church and do not always want to cremate the dead even in the twentieth century. Although, as we described in Chapter 5, the Western fear of death really began with the individual's self-awareness in the humanism movement of the twelfth century, and since then death has become an increasingly private matter, this privatization is not complete as long as people still gather together for funerals in church. The meeting there is undoubtedly an important social event, which, to some extent, gives people an opportunity to share the event of death.

With regard to contemporary Japanese society, the majority do not practise any religion, but they behave in a very traditional Shintoist or Buddhist way as will be remembered, for example in relation to 'the purification' that takes place in a modern hospital or after a funeral. The idea of 'giving oneself up into the fate of death' is still held by the Japanese patient and is in a way linked with both Shinto and Buddhist thought.   As Motoori Norinaga observed, in the Shinto philosophy (Chapter 6), death was to be absorbed in the world of the gods and we can be at peace by accepting death as a destiny which we have to become resigned to by harmonizing ourselves with the will of the gods. Or one of the most popular Japanese Buddhist sects like the Jodo sect (the Pure Land sect) teaches that by saying the name of 'Amida' we can be saved or go to the Pure Land. This idea seems to be based upon the belief in the inability of men to help themselves with regard to salvation and also to result from the need for practical and easy methods for salvation. We may have to reach this understanding before beginning to repeat the name of 'Amida' indicating that we are powerless before the coming of our death and therefore should accept it as a fate, in order to be able to rely on the mercy of 'Amida'. Here, we can again find the idea of 'giving up'. No matter whether in the Shinto or Buddhist belief, death seems to be inevitable and a part of the cosmic order or Nature. Even if people today do not practise either Shinto or Buddhism, their attitude to death and dying can therefore still correspond to the two religious traditions. Japanese people also gather together at religious funerals (following Buddhist ways in most cases), even if they do not usually get involved with the Buddhist faith. Thus we can find a strong link between the Japanese perspective on death and dying and their religious tradition in modern society. So, religions and religious rituals still have important values for modern Western and Japanese society, no matter whether people practise faith or not, and ritual seems to contribute to the possibility of sharing in the matter of death.

The Value of the Dead Body In Chapter 6 we discussed Japanese people's attachment to the dead bodies of their loved ones, in which dead bodies are not treated merely as things but still as persons as long as they have bodies which have not been cremated or buried. Even a dead body plays an important role in maintaining connections amongst members of the family or group. It seems to be too extreme to say that the West treats a dead body as a thing. Western people still often bury their loved ones' dead bodies without cremation as was mentioned in Chapter 5, and this is related to the Christian faith in the resurrection of the dead. Although the majority of Western people do not have faith in resurrection any more, they carry on burying corpses without cremating them, and this tells us that there is some residual value of the dead body or the idea of resurrection in the Western mind, which people are not necessarily aware of at a conscious level. Kubler-Ross says that an unhealthy grief and bereavement may remain in cases where one loses the opportunity to see the loved one's dead body, and does not participate in his burial (Kubler-Ross, 1983, p.70). Kubler-Ross also remarks that it is therapeutic for the dead person's relatives to keep the person's corpse in their house until the funeral, and that the family should be allowed to touch the dead person's body, for example, combing his hair (p.294). Kubler-Ross is a Swiss doctor practising in the United States, so her description is considered to be about American people and shows that there is such need for present day Americans. We could say that a dead body is not merely a thing for Western people, but something important in the process of accepting their loved ones' death, and that their notion of a dead body as being not only a thing is shared with Japanese people.

Differences

Changes in the Attitude to Death and Dying   In our consideration of similarities, we came to understand that there is a similar social climate surrounding the modern view of death, but we also need to recognize that the process involved before reaching this stage is different between the West and Japan. The West has changed its perspective on life and death gradually through the rise of individualism, the Enlightenment, the industrial revolution, and de-Christianization, all of which are related to one another. In a sense, therefore, the way death and dying are treated in modern Western society has arisen from this whole process. It has taken centuries for the current Western perspective on death and dying to emerge. Thus in the West, we can find a discontinuity between the old values such as death being shared by the community or the meaning of the Christian religion and the Christian community as a help for people to cope with death and bereavement, and the new values such as an emphasis on human rationality by which to think about the events of the world independently from God and so see man as a decision-maker having power over life and death, and regarding death and bereavement as taboo.

The Japanese modernization process has taken place only within the past fifty years or so. The high economic growth in the 1960s caused the structure of Japanese society to be remarkably urbanized and industrialized (Chapter 6) and Japanese medicine began to develop rapidly from this time. These two factors have had a strong influence on the way the Japanese die in this century which is similar to the process in the West mentioned early. The urbanization and industrialization of the country and the associated development of medicine can be attributed to the fact that Japan has imported Western technology, otherwise the speedy modernization and civilization, in less than a half century, would have been impossible. On the other hand, it is not realistic to imagine that the Japanese people's traditional ideas and thoughts built up in the past two thousand years could be washed away by Western ideas within such a short period.   How people die or how the dying are treated in contemporary Japanese society may be, in a sense, similar to the West, but at a deep level the Japanese attitude to death and dying is still traditional and basically has not changed since the third century, as we found when exploring the Japanese history of death and dying in Chapter 6. So, we may see a consistency in the Japanese attitude to death and dying at a deep level throughout centuries. The Japanese tradition and culture of death and dying seem to 'wear Western clothes' but under the Western clothes they have always been Japanese.

The change in the way Japanese people understand death seemed to occur suddenly but on the surface, while the Western change has occurred gradually taking place over hundreds of years and following the redefinition of the value of life and death in the Western mind.

Religious Tradition   Despite religious rituals remaining in the modern Western world, which play a certain role in people's sharing of the event of death, they do not seem to be a great help for people in coping with death and bereavement as we have indicated in Chapter 5. In the time before the de-Christianization of the eighteenth century, the Church community was at the centre of life, where the meaning of religion existed not only in rituals but in people's daily life, and people were bonded with each other by a strong tie. In the early Christian attitude to death and dying (Chapter 5), the whole community got involved with each person's death and dying, and the involvement remained even after the funeral or any other special occasions. On the other hand in the modern period, the meaning of religion as regards death seems to be very much limited to funerals, and the dead person's relatives are allowed to cry or to share matters of death with others mainly during the funeral. Visitors gathering together are often those who do not see each other except on this sort of occasion because, in urban society relatives and friends live far from each other, and are no longer part of the same village. Therefore, after the funeral, everyone has to go back to their own town, and the sharing and the bond between them during the funeral does not remain once the funeral is over; in other words, people close to the dead are normally left alone and are expected to 'pull themselves together' or act as if nothing had happened.

While religious tradition still remains in modern times, its meaning and effect are only apparent during the very short period of the funeral. This shortens the transition period from the time for mourning to the time for recovering and reintegrating into life, compared to the time before de-Christianization, when a person's death was an extended part of the life of the Christian community. In contemporary Western society, therefore it seems that Christian tradition and rituals may be becoming a small and disassociated part of an individual's life, which has some meaning and value only on special occasions like funerals and weddings.

We have explored in Chapter 5 that some religious symbolism remains even in secular Western minds, as found in the idea of 'bargaining' or the question of 'why me?' raised by the five stages proposed by Kubler-Ross in regard to dying patients. There must be some idea of God or supernatural authority as an object for their bargaining or questioning, though this does not mean patients are always fully conscious of it. The idea of a Christian God has been like 'buds of roses' in the deep dark forest of their hearts, and perhaps they have never been aware of it themselves nor has it any special influence on their moral judgments in their past life until the crisis of hearing the diagnosis of incurable disease. These forgotten 'roses', the idea of or some belief in God hidden within them, may suddenly flower in secularized Western people's minds at the time of their crisis and this may enable them to bargain or question. The 'roses' themselves, however, may be of such a nature that people may do these things without knowing where they want to address their bargaining or questioning or where such ideas come from in their mind. It looks as if the roses (the idea of a Christian God) within an individual have not been brought into their conscious mind by connecting them with religious faith, because what appears in their conscious mind is perhaps only 'the scent of roses' (religious values and symbolism without awareness of and conscious faith in God, e.g. symbolic ideas framed as the question 'why me?'). This may be why the meaning and effect of the Christian tradition are apparent only for the short period of the funeral. People's interests in practising religious rituals may be also 'the scent of roses' which has drifted only for a short period on special occasions.

In regard to Japan, as in the West, the majority do not practise any religion but participate in religious rituals only on special occasions. But the implication of this is different from in the West. Western de-Christianization has not only changed people's daily lives on the surface, but also their moral values, even if 'the scent of roses' is smelled only from time to time. People now see themselves as independent decision makers who can discern what is right or wrong for themselves. Although, the rise of this 'new' individualism would have been impossible without a background of Christian individualism and the humanism movement, the new individualism has changed the meaning and value of death and bereavement, and of religious rituals.

But in the case of the Japanese, it does not seem to make any great difference whether people practise religion or not as regards the meaning and value of death and bereavement. The Japanese have adjusted themselves to death and dying by accepting them in resignation to a fate to be sad about throughout the centuries and even down to the modern period of the twentieth century. As seen in exploring similarities, these ideas are strongly linked with the Shinto and Buddhist traditions. The two religions might not be practised as religions by the majority of Japanese people any more but remain as philosophies in their mind. So, as in the West, the idea of God or a supernatural power within the unconscious mind of modern Japanese people might be also like the 'hidden roses' in the Western mind (though they are not the same flowers as 'roses' because of their different religious tradition). But their 'scent' tends to fill their whole life, while appearing only on special occasions for modern Western people. The religious values are still reflected in the ordinary Japanese life, and the modern Japanese attitude to life, human relationships, and death and dying remains, therefore, at a deep level, very much Shintoist or Buddhist.

It may be Japanese culture itself which has created and arranged the two religions suitable for itself. For instance, in the case of the Pure Land sect of popular Japanese Buddhism, the Japanese produced the easiest methods of salvation for the lay public. The fact that these easiest and practical methods became popular amongst the Japanese can be related to the nature of the Japanese mind. This suggests that Japanese people already had the essential nature of the religion (e.g. Japanese people's practical nature) before the religion appeared. Thus, we are not sure whether the Japanese people created their religions as appropriate for themselves, or the religions have had an influence on the Japanese personality. Both are probably involved and this unclear 'chicken and egg' situation itself explains the reason why the 'scent' of Buddhism and Shinto (their religious values without conscious faith in them), continuously fills (having an influence on) modern Japanese people's lives and their moral values. So, the West and Japan may appear similar in the fact that religious rituals still remain even in the modern period, but the meaning in the two cases needs to be distinguished.

Individuality and Death   We have accepted in our investigation of similarities that death is not an event only of an individual but of society both in contemporary Western as well as Japanese society. It is, however, necessary to see a distinction between 'a social event' in an individualistic society and in a non- or less individualistic one. For example, respect for the dead body is, to some extent, considered to be present in the modern West and Japan as we have seen earlier, but the underlying meaning of the same tendency can be different between the two. Kubler-Ross points out that a dead body is merely a shell or cocoon of the person (Kubler-Ross, 1983, p.292), but for Western people the shell or the cocoon should not be treated in just the same way as rubbish. We may be able to use the word 'an extended self' for the dead body. Suppose, when you are walking a dog and someone says 'He is lovely!', you feel good as if you yourself were thought of as a lovely person because the dog is your 'extended self' and you have a strong identification of your self-respect with the dog. A dead body might be also considered as 'an extended self' of the dead person, and this may be why Western people respect or treat it carefully.

We would hypothesize that Western people identify the dead person with his body but not themselves with the dead or his body, because in their ordinary life, an individual ego or self is to be distinguished from that of others. Even the Christian idea of 'denying yourself' seems to imply the existence of an individual self, and it would be impossible to do this if there were no such existence of a 'self'. A strong awareness of an individual self within a Western person may prevent identification with the dead person or his body, as it does with other living people.

Japanese people may, however, identify with a dead body not as a cocoon or a dead person's 'extended self' but almost as a living person. In a less individualistic society, with a lack of self-awareness throughout history, and a homogeneous culture, the Japanese have not drawn a clear line between themselves and others though they may have done so between their community and other communities. As we have explained in Chapters 3 and 6, important decisions in an individual Japanese person's life tend to be made by or with his family or the people in his community. Therefore individual responsibility for death and disease is not strong. To lose someone has a big effect on the rest of the community, but this does not only mean to lose the person but to lose a part of each member's existential value and this may explain the Japanese difficulty in accepting others' deaths and their attachment to dead relatives' bodies.

The dead person and his dead body may appear to be identified in Japan as in the West, but the meaning is different from the West, because they are identified not as if the dead body is 'a cocoon' or 'an extended ego' of the dead person, but as a living person, who has been related to the existential value of each member of the community. The identification amongst people in the Japanese community with their lack of self-awareness may make one person's death their own death. But in fact they are still alive and therefore need to have a certain period of time for treating the dead body as a living person until the cremation of the body, when they and their community begin to redefine and reestablish the value and meaning of the community without the dead and so 'resurrect' themselves. There may be some similar cases where Western people treat a dead person as still living, and where the difference becomes smaller than is suggested here, but usually they are supposed to distinguish themselves from the dead.

Sad and Frightening Deaths We need first to clarify that we are talking about 'death' but not 'dying', which implies the dying process and could be an object of fear for people in both the modern West and Japan because of dehumanization in the modern hospital. We have explained that one of the important aspects of the Japanese attitude to death is the idea of a 'sad death', which can be compared with the Western 'fear of death'. It is incorrect to say that there is no fear of death in the Japanese mind, however 'sadness' may still be a crucial aspect of the way in which the Japanese perceive death. It is possible to fear the cause of 'sadness' but at the same time we may see the Japanese accepting death (the cause of sadness) by being sad about it, rather than fearing it, when we consider Japanese passivity in accepting death and disease as a fate not to be fought against. In the long feudal period with its lack of self-awareness, an individual's life and death were affected by the destiny of his community, so an individual had no choice except accepting his fate so that he could be loyal to his community. This sharing of the fate of death, on the other hand, must have reduced the fear of death because of the recognition of death as an event and a fate of the whole community.

If one fears death as the cause of one's sadness, one may begin to take a certain action in order to change the frightening situation, or even if that person is not aware of his fear of something, he may sometimes take an action unconsciously in order to avoid the situation in self-defence. Even if avoiding a frightening condition is a cowardly action, it is still considered to be an active reaction to fight against the situation rather than just to accept it. The attempt to avoid or change the frightening situation is an active approach, which needs to be distinguished from just accepting it or giving it up as a sad fate. It seems that death is to be accepted as a sad thing, but not as an object to fight against for Japanese people. As we described in Chapter 6, sadness is often linked with the object of compassion. When one becomes sad on hearing about a best friend being depressed about her mother's death, this sadness is not an enemy to conquer or fight against. Even the cause of the sadness, the friend's mother's death may not be the object of fear but of sadness in the Japanese mind, though, for Japanese people, accepting others' deaths seems to be more difficult than accepting their own death. We should emphasize again that it is too extreme to say that the Japanese do not fear death at all or could not experience both fear and sadness at the same time, but that it is still important to notice their passive attitude to death and disease which fits the description of a 'sad death' more easily than a 'frightening death'.

On the other hand, since about the twelfth century, the Western world has had a long history of the fear of death and fighting against it. In Western history, the fear before de-Christianization was caused by the idea of the Last Judgment, strengthened particularly from the twelfth century by the rise of individualism. The fear arose after de-Christianization occurred, in the modern age after the time of the Enlightenment, by the fact that death became 'a dead line' which destroys an individual's aspiration, self-esteem, and self-actualization, through the privatization of death and related emotional issues. The Enlightenment encouraged an individual to control his life by himself independent from God or any other religious authorities. Before de-Christianization, with a strengthened awareness of an individual self, people had become conscious of their own death and the Last Judgment. As we mentioned in Chapter 4, pilgrimages and hospices had become popular from this period (the twelfth century), and this may show that people tried to overcome their fear of the Last Judgment and death by taking pilgrimages to Shrines and gaining forgiveness of sin. The rational secular ideas of the Enlightenment encouraged people's ability to control their own lives without a religious faith, so the Christian faith began to decline. Medical science emerged from this period and started on the long process of attempting to conquer death, which takes away peoples' freedom to achieve, to fulfil, and to enjoy all happiness and pleasures in life. Both before and after de-Christianization, therefore, the West has tried to control and overcome death, by pilgrimages in former times and medical science latterly, and the fear of death, seems to exist behind each approach to some extent.

An important point here is that what this 'active approach' is directed towards is different before and after de-Christianization. Formerly it was a way of accepting physical death and conquering spiritual death by repentance (e.g. through taking pilgrimages), and eventually it may have reduced the fear of physical death because this was in part related to the fear of spiritual death through its association with the faith in the Last Judgment and hell. Physical death itself was still of course frightening for people, but perhaps more frightening for those who had a strong Christian faith, may have been 'spiritual death' represented in the idea of eternal punishment. On the other hand, the latter situation tries to conquer the fear of physical death alone by intensive medical treatments and technologies, which aim to fight against and deny physical death. The acceptance of physical death found in former times, however, must not be equated with the Japanese acceptance of death. The Western acceptance in the time before de-Christianization needed special 'work and effort' such as prayers, pilgrimages, atonement of sins, etc, as the idea of 'taking up one's own cross' implies, and as a result of which people can feel peace (as they feel themselves able to go to heaven) and accept their own physical death more easily. To the extent that there was an awareness of an individual self, it was still possible to control one's situation (e.g. whether or not one wants to go to hell after death). Even if one's whole family are destined to go to hell, there is still a chance of repentance through one's own 'work and effort'! This has to be separated from the Japanese acceptance of physical death by 'giving up the situation' without making any such special effort, because a Japanese individual's destiny is not up to his own effort or decisions but has been deeply influenced by the group he belongs to, as seen in the destiny of the warrior (Chapter 6). There is no active attitude to death involved, and that is why death is something one can only be sad about in the Japanese mind.

It is wrong to say that people in the West never feel sad about death, but an important distinction to be made between the Western and the Japanese attitude is that the West has had a tendency to try to change or fight against the situation which will cause sadness until reaching the stage in which there was nothing to do but be sad about it. This is not the same as the Japanese tendency of just giving up or accepting fate. The relatively active approach to death in the West found in its history will be more likely to lead to the idea of a 'frightening death', since, as we mentioned earlier, the object of fear is often deeply related to the notion of an 'enemy'. It is of course possible to be fearful and sad at the same time or one can be sad because of fear. Suppose, you are confronted by a murderer, who looks physically much stronger than you, and you cry because of fear. At the point of your crying, however, you are more likely to be out of control and so are passive; in other words, you may not attempt to fight against the person. What is suggested by this example is that sadness is more likely to imply a sort of passivity towards the situation, and the Western history of conquering death, whether spiritual or physical, might have been impossible if the idea of death had been merely of a sad matter, but the alternative a long existing fear of death might have made death a challenge.

In regard to the five psychological stages introduced by Kubler-Ross, we are not certain now that her idea, even if it may sometimes be appropriate for Western people, is also so for Japanese people. We suggested in Chapter 5 that the fear of death reinforced the first four stages: denial and isolation, anger, bargaining, and depression, or was the background to them. We may not be able to apply this to Japanese people though, because they have not had a strong fear of death but mainly accepted it by 'giving in to fate'.

Attitudes to Suicide and Voluntary Active Euthanasia Japanese culture has not had the notion of eternal punishment or of suicide as a deadly sin as interpreted in the Christian doctrine. In fact, Japanese Buddhist monks found it hard to understand the idea of eternal punishment in Christianity, though they seemed to easily accept Christian altruism and the emphasis on love. Death has tended to be something sad for Japanese people, which is connected to the object of compassion. Killing oneself because of unendurable pain or to avoid shame may be also the subject of compassion and mercy. But historically suicide has been unforgivable for the Western mind following the long Christian tradition, which insists that only God has authority over human life so humans have no right to abandon it by their own will. But, since de-Christianization began in the West from the eighteenth century, man started to replace God and insist on his right to be the author of his own life, deciding the meaning and the value of life so that he can have the right to end life if it does not have meaning or good quality as defined by himself but is full of uncontrollable pain. Such ideas make the acceptance of voluntary active euthanasia possible.

As to Japan, although it has a relatively tolerant attitude towards suicide, voluntary active euthanasia is not considered seriously even in the Japan Society for Dying with Dignity, which is more interested in spreading Living Wills throughout society. It may be difficult for a Japanese person to insist on his right to die considering his lack of self-awareness in daily life. If an act of active euthanasia were to take place, it might well be the family who asked the doctor to do it for the patient's good. In Japanese history, suicide of warriors has been taken for granted, however, their suicide was strongly connected with their community and Lord to whom they swore their loyalty. They had to die (as mentioned in Chapter 6) in order to avoid their enemies killing them or living in shame as a loser, but such suicidal acts were not the result of an individual's awareness of his life but of the group's. The Japanese may die in relation to their community, superiors, and so on, but not die as an individual even in the case of suicide. So, the idea of voluntary active euthanasia is not consonant with the Japanese attitude to suicide, even though on the surface it looks similar, because the former is impossible without an individual awareness of the right to control one's own life and death, but in the latter, in most cases, individuals had to kill themselves as acceptance of the inevitable destiny of their community. To some extent, therefore, the concept of 'voluntary' does not accord with Japanese culture since the word requires one to claim the rights of an individual.

Attitudes to Death and Dying, and the Hospice Movement in a Comparison between the West and Japan

In the first section of this chapter, we have made a comparison between the Western and the Japanese attitude to death and dying, and discovered similarities and differences. We will now look at this work together with that on the hospice movement in the West and Japan, which we analyzed Part I of the book, to see how the different attitudes to death and dying are connected with the hospice movement in Japan and the West in order to glimpse what sort of problems Japan may have in attempting to import the Western hospice and its philosophy.

Religious Tradition

We explored in Chapter 5 how the Western hospice has attempted to revive the early Christian attitude to death and dying, in which individuals could prepare for a predicted death, have faith in and hope for resurrection, no strong awareness of the Last Judgment, and see death and bereavement as an event of the whole community. We have also explored the possibility that the modern hospice may create these conditions, by means of a modern 'pilgrimage' in order to overcome the fear of death and dying, no longer arising through an awareness of the Last Judgment but from the secularized way of life which regards death as a mere dead line, the modern taboo on emotional issues, the development of medical science, etc. On the other hand, however, we have seen that such a 'revival' has only been developed in a sense as part of the problems of hospice care, observing that the public attitude to death and bereavement is still not at all open although there has been great financial support for the hospice movement.

Coming back to the 'rose' analogy, we may say that the modern hospice movement may intend to use the 'scent of roses', religious values and symbolism, which have remained in the modern secularized Western mind and without an awareness of God's existence, in order to complete the pilgrim-cancer patient metaphor. In the change of moral values resulting from the secularization of Western life and thought, the 'scent of roses' may, as we have seen, only become apparent on special occasions such as funerals, weddings, and crises of people's lives, but not in the ordinary daily life of the modern period. We suppose that is why it has been necessary to create another world called the 'hospice', which by analogy may be described as a 'greenhouse', in order to revive the old Christian perspective on death and dying or 'pilgrimage' within certain limits under the hospice philosophy.

For the Japanese, ordinary modern life is, compared to the West, full of 'scent'. That is to say, the scent is not only for special occasions, and this is because people's day-to-day attitudes to life, death, and human relationships are deeply influenced by religious values though they are not practising traditional religions like Shinto and Buddhism. But the scent comes from different sorts of flowers, for example 'lilies', because of its different religious tradition from the Western one. However Japanese palliative care units are deeply linked with the Western hospice movement, whose strong Christian background is not familiar to the majority of the lay public. So, as in the West, it may be difficult to develop the Western notion of 'hospice care' except through creating a 'special space'. This special space is, however, not a 'greenhouse', since the greenhouse analogy in the Western situation implies the existence of 'the wasteland', which is outside hospice care where death and emotional issues are not accepted by the public. There is no 'wasteland' in the Japanese situation in regard to the Japanese attitude to death and dying, which is communal and does not involve a strong fear of death.

Building 'greenhouses' in the West may be easier than the 'special spaces' in Japan, because the former revives an old Christian attitude while the latter adds new religious (Christian) values to the old traditional religious (Shinto and Buddhist) values in order to change the old into the new. In the modern secularized Western mind, there has been the 'scent of roses' wafting around at least on special occasions, and if you walk towards where the 'scent' comes from, its origin may eventually be traced to the 'roses themselves', which are faith in God and the old Christian attitude to life, death and dying. In the Japanese case, however, to build 'special spaces' based on the borrowed idea of the Western hospice means to plant a rose bush for the first time, while only 'lilies' (Buddhism and Shinto) have been grown there before.

With regard to the idea of 'pilgrimage', it may be difficult for the majority of Japanese cancer patients and their families to understand or accept such an idea by means of which people can overcome the fear of death. The reason is that the Japanese have not really had any significant experience of fighting against death or trying to overcome it through fear, but have tended to accept it more passively as a natural cause of sadness. The idea of 'shouldering one's own cross and following Christ' on a pilgrimage is an active reaction to life and death, which respects the meaning and responsibility for life (the cross) of each individual so that he walks carrying the cross to overcome fear and sin actively. Japanese incurable cancer patients, however, who do not know the nature of their disease and are normally brought to the hospice by their families, are not able to make such a pilgrimage. The idea of a 'sad death' in the Japanese mind does not lend itself to the Western hospice notion of 'pilgrimage'.

It is not realistic to imagine that the Japanese passive attitude of a 'sad death' will be able to change suddenly into the Christian active approach towards death and dying, because the Japanese outlook as represented in the concept of a 'sad death' has existed at a very deep level in the Japanese mind throughout centuries, as we described in Chapter 6. No matter how much people are modernized and stop practising traditional religions like Shinto and Buddhism, which are deeply related to the idea of a 'sad death' and passivity towards events of this world, religious values themselves have remained active in the ordinary Japanese mind.

Another possibility is that the fear of death may begin to grow in the Japanese mind, where it did not exist significantly before, if Japan attempted to establish hospices so as to organize 'pilgrimages' to overcome the 'fear of death'. It would be paradoxical as well as ironic if the Japanese people were forced to 'fear' death by introducing the Western hospice, which has aimed to conquer the fear of death.

The Image of the Hospice

In Chapter 6 we explored how the hospice may have the image of the 'dirtiest place' in the future because of the Japanese image of disease and death as 'dirt' and of the original meaning of the Japanese word 'byo-in' (a house surrounded by a wall to separate disease). Palliative care units for incurable cancer patients could be seen as the dirtiest places in this sense. But as we mentioned in Chapter 2, the word 'hospice' has not been associated with any such negative sense but with that of 'guest' or 'hospitality' or a 'stranger' to be treated kindly and respected as with Jesus. It may be, however, hard for the Japanese to envisage giving hospitality to 'Christ' inside the same building as 'a house to separate disease' or a 'dirty place' without changing the whole notion of 'hospital' and of 'death and disease' as 'dirt'.

PART III
THE DOCTOR-PATIENT RELATIONSHIP AND THE HOSPICE MOVEMENT

8 Doctors, Patients, and the Western Hospice Movement

Introduction

In the first section of this chapter, we will explore how the role of the doctor has been understood; how society has perceived the doctor; and what sort of relationship the doctor and the patient have had. This will help us to see one of the aspects which the hospice philosophy has tried to counter, that is, the nature of human relationships in hospitals. In the second section, we will discuss the connection between the doctor-patient relationship and the hospice movement, together with our observations from the preceding chapter on the hospice and attitudes to death and dying.

The Western Doctor-Patient Relationship

The Mask of the Doctor

A human relationship between two persons is an interaction between them, an important aspect being whether one person has more authority than the other person does; or one has a stronger influence on the relationship than the other does. Western doctors have worn different 'masks' to play different roles in dealing with their patients, but the question is who made these masks. In a famous play based upon the story of Pygmalion written by Bernard Shaw, there is a scene in which Eliza, the heroine of the story, says:

> [T]he difference between a lady and a flower girl is not how she behaves, but how she's treated. I shall always be a flower girl to Professor Higgins, because he always treats me as a flower girl, and always will; but I know I can be a lady to you, because you always treat me as a lady, and always will. (Shaw, 1992, pp.93-95)

Interestingly there might be a point at which she can no longer remember whether being a 'lady' is a mask or her real nature. When she is treated and behaves as a lady feeling comfortable being so, she might forget the fact that at the beginning she was asked to wear a mask. Or she might no longer be anything else even if she takes the mask off; that is to say, to be a lady is not a role to perform any longer but becomes part of her own personality. We could never be certain, however, that 'the mask of a lady' was created only by others rather than Eliza herself. In other words, it might be possible that 'the seed of a lady' within Eliza could be made to flower by people who treat her as a lady, and that means she already had the innate nature to be a lady since the time when she used to be a flower girl or to speak English with a cockney accent. This can be distinguished from making her have the external appearance of a 'lady' by the manner in which she is treated, but the story does not clarify in which way (or in both ways) Eliza was transformed. But it is possible to say at least that she was given a mask of a lady in the beginning and this mask had an influence on her personality whether it was because the mask reminded her of her innate lady's nature or changed her personality completely from a flower girl into a lady.

The doctors' 'mask' might be considered in a similar way to Eliza's case. It might be said that society or patients have created certain images of the doctor. Sometimes the doctor is almost forced to wear 'the masks' by society or patients in order to play expected roles, but at other times the doctor might feel comfortable with the masks which may benefit him in some ways, and forget the fact that he is wearing masks. The doctor no longer remembers who created the masks because the masks are becoming one with his own face; in other words, the masks have a strong influence on his personality and his way of behaving even outside his medical practice. So while doctors begin by wearing masks they tend to become merged with their own faces. In order to understand the Western doctor-patient relationship, the idea of doctor's masks is a very important aspect to look at, since this has had an influence on the relationship. There are many 'masks' of the doctor, but we will consider two of them here, which are often linked with problems of the doctor-patient relationship. The first tends to exist symbolically, and the second seems to be still significant literally in modern Western societies.

The Doctor as a Priest/Father The physician is like a priest to some extent and the analogy seems to be derived from the Hippocratic phrase 'In purity and holiness I will practice my art'. In this idea, the physician is expected to have two kinds of desire: philatechnian, love of technique;

and philanthropia, love of persons, both of which are congruent with the nature of the priesthood (Vaux, 1988, pp.128-130).

The idea of vocation The image of the priesthood reminds us of the idea of vocation, which leads us to feel that priests are people chosen by God as the Hippocratic phrase 'purity and holiness' implies. We are not certain whether every doctor can develop the image of a priest and father, in the way that Eliza saw herself as becoming a lady through being treated as one. There might be some necessary quality of the individual by which he or she *deserves* to receive the mask of a priest, and this idea can be connected with that of vocation. Being a 'doctor' is to have a job but must be distinguished from any other job, as is the priesthood, because the doctor may be 'chosen' or 'called' to be a doctor. Where does such an idea come from? First of all, we need to remember some expectations about physicians, which have been universal throughout history; to be a genuinely caring person who can deal with the difficult situation of the patient, and also to have special knowledge to do so (Van Eys, 1988, p.13).

'Caring' and 'love' are often parallels, and indeed, 'Paracelsus recognized a special dedication and commitment that characterized art when he said, 'Where there is no love there is no art'' (Van Eys, 1988, p.7). Erich Fromm also says in his 'The Art of Loving' that love is to care for someone as much as oneself (Fromm, 1956; cited by Van Eys, 1988, pp.7-8). In their love and caring, priests have to guide people to God through salvation; heal the sick; and give absolution to repentant sinners, and all this is made possible through a special relationship with God. In Christianity, Jesus Christ is understood to accomplish miracles to cure the sick not by his own will but in a perfect faith in and obedience with God's will. Likewise, in the image of the doctor as a priest, his treatment and healing of the patient are considered to be done through the intervention of God.

This special relationship between God and the doctor might be recognized in the concept 'physiophiloa' (love of nature) of the Hippocratic Oath in which doctors are required to show humility towards nature (Knight, 1988, pp.31-32). 'Love of Nature' or 'humility towards Nature' may be seen as corresponding to love and humility towards God as the creator of Nature. Becoming humble before God or Nature, the doctor can cooperate appropriately with God and heal people in need. So the word 'love' can have a spiritual or religious implication; that is to say, love is related to God. All sorts of jobs which involve 'caring for others' or 'loving others' could be thought of as sacred jobs because they are done in relationship with God; in other words, priests and doctors may be considered as partners of God. The doctor's image as a partner of God can then create the sacred image of the doctor. With regard to the partnership, as one chooses a partner for his or her married life, so does God with some people in the idea of vocation. Coming back to the case of Eliza in Pygmalion which we discussed earlier, we can connect the doctor's vocation with the innate nature of a lady within Eliza. The doctor might be considered as a person who has some inherent nature for which God chooses him and for which he deserves 'the mask of the doctor'. Where a belief in this innate nature is held, it will strengthen the sacred image of the doctor.

Although we have seen the underlying notion of the priest-mask of the doctor, Western society and medicine are very much secularized now, so most people no longer see the doctor as a partner of God as with a priest, but the symbolic imagery may still remain. Science has contributed to keeping this image of the doctor, because it is becoming the replacement for God and people may regard the doctor as a partner of a new 'God' named 'science', or 'a priest', who can use a 'magic cure' (scientific technologies) and has close contact with the world of 'God' (science). Here, we can see a parallel between the doctor's image as a priest and as a scientist, and we will explore the connection between the doctor and science later.

The idea of 'father' Fatherhood is 'an alternative symbol for the priestly model', since "father' has traditionally been a personalistic metaphor for God and for the priest' (Veatch, 1991, p.13). The idea of the doctor as a priest or father seems to be the source of doctors' paternalism. The Hippocratic Oath ' ... according to my ability and judgment, I consider for the benefit of my patients ... ' (cited by Veatch, p.35) has been regarded as the origin of doctors' paternalism in modern medical ethics in the West. Medical professionals have repeatedly used this idea in the ethical code in past centuries. The Hippocratic principles tend to permit the physician's paternalistic behaviour as far as, from the physician's point of view, it is considered to benefit the patient no matter whether or not the patient accepts it (Veatch, 1991, pp.63-65). Many physicians in the modern period still think that they are entitled to have the authority to make medical decisions (Sherwin, 1992, p.139).

The origin of the word 'doctor' is the Latin 'docere' which means 'to teach' (*An Etymological Dictionary of the English Language*). The image of a teacher overlaps with that of a father, who may bring about changes within the child. A father has an authority to make important decisions for his children, and traditionally his children must both fear him and be obedient to him. The patient may also have fear of this kind of the doctor; for example, many patients feel anxiety in meeting their doctors as the following quotation from a patient shows:

> Patients get tensed up waiting. If you could just walk in it would be better but the patients all sit in rows and say 'Is he in a good mood today?' (DHSS, 1979, p.38)

A father's authority is sometimes one-sided as when we find that God asks Abraham to make Isaac, his only son, a sacrifice for God (Genesis 22), where no questioning of God's behest is permitted. Patients may find it difficult to question their doctors as father figures and physicians rarely explain what patients want or need to know, as research shows that doctors spend less than one percent of the total time of their meetings with patients in explanations to them (Wallen, *et al.*, 1979; cited by West, 1983, p.75). In the Western doctor-patient relationship, the doctor tends to play the role of questioner and the patient, the role of answerer.

The Doctor as a Scientist and Technician Science has had a strong influence on the modern image of doctors and the development of doctors' social status. We will consider how doctors' status has developed in history, taking the example of British doctors.

The history of doctors' social status Medical education in Oxford University had already begun in the ninth century and became well established by the twelfth century, however, medicine was understood as an intellectual rather than a practical activity, and reasoning was considered most important. The physician sometimes just gave a written opinion or advice to the patient without seeing him or her, and was regarded as an educated person who should not be put in the humble position of dirtying his hands by performing operations or touching the bodies of patients. All dirty jobs were done by the apothecaries, and the barber-surgeons. The apothecaries were naturally connected with medicine because of their dealing with herbs, spices, and the corpses of animals, etc, and also imported drugs and fragments of human mummies. The barber-surgeons were barbers as well as undertaking medical surgery. These people carrying out the practical side of medicine were lower in social status than the physicians who worked on the academic side. Until the nineteenth century, the role of the professional had the image of a 'gentleman' who was not supposed to do any manual labour (Bennet,

1987, pp.47-62).

From the time of the Enlightenment in the middle of the eighteenth century, the law gave surgeons their own company, and surgery was developed significantly by the late eighteenth century, reflecting the emergence of science and its technological development in the medical field. Science changed the image of the professional from a person dealing with a purely theoretical study into one involving both theory and practice. It was at this time that John Hunter (1728-93) rationalized surgery. Through his great contribution, surgeons started their own Royal College, where their skills were developed rapidly, and they had the prestige and economic power to become respectable figures. Thereafter the social standing of the surgeon soon became as high as the physician, perceived as a professional man, and since then to the present day the surgeon and the physician have both been powerful within medicine (Bennet, 1987, p.53).

We have seen then that, under the influence of science since the Enlightenment, surgeons have been accepted into the world of professionals and the intelligentsia together with physicians, and both surgeons and physicians are now regarded as 'the doctor' who deals with both theory and practice.

Science and the doctor - medical education Cassell observes of medical students that 'despite the many different countries in which they receive their medical education, they are all trained in essentially the same manner as the American student' (Cassell, 1978, p.85). (We may better understand Cassell's expression 'many different countries' as civilized countries in the East and the West.) This is because all medical schools in the different countries of the Western world are likely to concentrate on objective, technical, and scientific aspects of medicine but disregard the aspects in which social sciences and humanities are involved (Sherwin, 1992, p.146). Scientific description refers to the description of only measurable quantities such as temperature but not of anything qualitative, and scientific method is more concerned with generality than individuality (Cassell, 1991, p.18).

Science and the doctor - scientific objectivity and the doctor-patient relationship With the emphasis on scientific objectivity, doctors are not expected to have an emotional involvement with their patients, but ought to be detached from them (Veatch, 1991, p.34). Hence, 'medical students and junior doctors may be criticized for being 'emotional' and failing to maintain 'true scientific objectivity'' (Bennet, 1987, p.164). This denial of emotions in all of medicine has led the doctor to deny the patient's emotions. Recently patients have begun to complain about the doctor's treatment of them merely as objects and not as humans with emotions, as the following quotations show:

> He didn't tell me anything. Just gave me the prescription. He's writing out the prescription as he's talking to you. He just doesn't seem to listen. (DHSS, 1979, p.58)

> The doctor's just like a machine working to time. (*ibid.* p.38).

> The doctor just looks at you as if you were a number. (*ibid.*)

> I object very strongly to being a number in a book. You're no longer a person these days. (*ibid.*)

Science and the doctor - the sacred world of the doctor as a scientist
The image of medicine as scientific tends to 'persuade both doctors and patients that medicine is a complex field and that medical decision-making involves a level of understanding far beyond the reach of nonspecialists (Shorter, 1985; cited by Sherwin, 1992, p.146). This tends to fortify the paternalism of the doctor by letting him hide away in 'the sacred world' called medical science into which others are forbidden to enter. We have seen that modern Western society does not always look at the doctor as being in the image of a priest or a partner with God any more but the symbolic image has remained. Such religious symbolism and authority seem to have been taken over by the doctor as a partner of 'new God' (science) in the 'sacred' world of medical science.

The Complexity of the Relationship between the Nature of the Masks and the Doctor

Although we have looked at two masks of the doctor, as a priest or father and a scientist, it is necessary to understand the complicated nature of the relationship between the masks and the doctor in order to avoid an oversimplification in the perception of the notion of 'the doctor'.

The Mysterious Power of Masks We have seen that some doctors emerged from the practical aspect of medicine, for example barber-surgeons who began to raise their social status as they absorbed scientific technologies for treating diseases. That is to say, the mask of a scientist helped them to improve their social standing. But the mask does not work in a straightforward way, because even if a worker making a car in a factory learns scientific methods to make or repair cars, his social status will remain that of the working class. The same can be said with the mask of a priest and a father. For example, a Eucharistic minister may begin to distribute the Eucharist in the Catholic Church, which used to be done only by priests, but a Eucharistic minister cannot have the same authority as priests have in giving a sacrament of penance. The mask of a priest, a father, or a scientist does not always work for every wearer in the same way as it does for the doctor, and we may find that there is a mysterious way in which the masks work only when the doctor uses them. It may be like Excalibur, which could be pulled out from a great stone only by King Arthur. Thus a secret of the magical power of the masks is hidden not only in the masks themselves but also in the doctor who wears them or in the interaction between the doctor and the masks. So the concept of 'the doctor' must be understood not in the nature of the masks alone but in the nature of the interaction between the doctor and the masks as well. Therefore, the notion of 'the doctor' is complicated and cannot be defined only by one of the roles of the masks as those of a priest or father and a scientist. The doctor cannot be a real priest because his patients are not his congregation; nor can he be a real father because his patients are not his children; nor wholly a scientist because his patients are not merely objects for scientific experiments. Even if these masks are integrated and become one mask, this is not sufficient to express the complete role or notion of the doctor unless we can discover the factor that produces 'a magical power' in the interaction between the doctor and the masks. While the masks which we have discussed are a very important part of the nature of the doctor's role because many problems in the doctor-patient relationship are often concerned with them, the complexity of the doctor's masks requires further consideration in relation to 'magical power' and this will be considered later.

Different Expectations of Masks It may be that the patient's complaints as discussed under the heading of The Mask of the Doctor are all related to the nature of the doctor's mask (as a priest/father and scientist), but on the other hand, the patient, to some extent, still seems to expect the doctor to have the image of a priest as well as a scientist who has great authority. An interesting gap between the doctor and the patient in terms of their attitudes to the mask is that the doctor sometimes wears the mask of a priest/father and scientist in a way the patient does not approve of, and that the doctor does not always wear them in the way convenient for the patient. Such expressions by the patient as we saw in the preceding section (for example 'The doctor just looks at you as if you were a number') may show that patients want to be cared for and be treated as human by the doctor, and to be treated in this way could be seen as a part of the doctor's mask as a priest/father. Also, many people, especially the young, expect a more friendly approach from the doctor, but they also want a businesslike and technically skilled doctor (DHSS, 1979, p.85), and this may require the mask of the doctor as a scientist. The distance between what the doctor is doing and what the patient expects the doctor to do in relation to the two masks might be explained by different expectations of the masks between them. The doctor may use the masks to benefit himself as well as the patient, but the patient may think of the masks as being used only for the patient's benefit. The doctor himself might not be aware of whether he behaves paternalistically because of his desire to defend himself from stress and anxiety or protect the patient from anxiety or achieve successful medical results for his own credit. The crucial point here is, however, that the masks may be acknowledged by both doctors and patients, but the expectations of the masks may be very different between them.

An Interaction between Masks We need to understand also that the masks of the doctor are not completely independent from one another, because they are interacting. For instance, the modern doctor as a scientist may be symbolically 'sacred' like a priest because he has special and exclusive knowledge about scientific technologies and may use this 'healing magic' efficiently.

Vulnerable Doctors

There must be a possibility that because of one's scientific ability or priestlike caring nature one could become a doctor by getting through all sorts of difficult training, education, and examinations, but it is also possible that one becomes increasingly professionalised as a doctor by wearing the masks of a scientist and a priest, so playing certain expected roles in society. No matter whether or not these 'scientific' and 'priest-like' natures constitute the genuine personality of an individual who wants to be a doctor, a vulnerable face as a human beneath the masks must be considered an important condition for a healer. Carl Jung says that only the wounded person can heal because he is open and sensitive about another person's pain and suffering so that he is able to take part in healing the person (Jung, 1954; cited by Knight, 1988, p.33). Healing activities are connected with the human vulnerability of the healer and the patient (Nowwen, 1972; cited by Knight, 1988, p.33).

Both Jung and Nowwen seem to think that one who knows his own vulnerability and weakness could understand another person's pain; and that this understanding could heal the person. To understand one's own vulnerability and hurt may lead one to reach the knowledge of how to deal with, care for, and heal one's own wound. But if one does not try to understand and care about his own weakness and wound, it will become 'a volcano' of his repressed emotion and stress, which may erupt and destroy his life in the end. The modern doctor may be 'a wounded healer' who does not know his own wound. Coming back to the mysterious power in the doctor's interaction with the two masks, we may be able to bring in the idea of a healer here. The reason why the mask of a priest and a scientist has such strength particularly for the doctor, might be that he wears the mask of a healer also and the two other masks interact with the healer's mask, so that magical power is created in the interaction. Taking the idea of a 'wounded healer', we may say that whether the interaction occurs for the benefit of the patient or the doctor himself or both, may be related, to some extent, to whether the doctor knows his vulnerable face as a human underneath the masks. Before thinking more about his wound, let us first consider some defensive attitudes of the doctor in relation to the matter of death.

Defensive Attitudes of the Doctor   Here we will consider the doctor as a bad listener, and doctors' fears.

The doctor as a bad listener   We have already discussed how physicians are likely to ask questions and patients to respond in their conversation. Also, patients often use terms such as 'yeah', 'uh huh', and 'yep' in answering the doctor's questions, which tend to show acknowledgement, agreement and understanding of another person's statement (West, 1983, p.79). Why the conversation is onesided may not be only because the doctor does not have enough time for listening to each of his patients, but may also be because the doctor tries to reduce the opportunity to answer or listen to what he does not want to hear, such as matters of death or painful personal issues. This is illustrated in the dialogues between the doctor and the patient detailed in the next section, where we can see the doctor's defensive attitude to the patient.

Doctors' fears   People's defensive attitudes can be related to certain kinds of fear, and the doctor's defence mechanism emerges from at least two of them. Firstly, the doctor fears the issue of death and emotion; secondly, the risk of making mistakes in his medical practice. We can find the doctor's fear of death in the following dialogues between the doctor and the patient:

(1)

Surgeon: Well, how are you today?

Woman (dying of breast cancer): I'm very worried about what is happening to me. I'm beginning to think I'm not going to get better this time. The pain in my hip is getting worse.

Surgeon: Tell me more about this pain in your hip.

(2)

Doctor: How are you today?

Patient (dying of lung cancer): I'm not too good. I can't understand why I'm continuing to lose so much weight.

Doctor: Have you had any pain?

Patient: I'm not going to get out of here, am I?

Doctor: Have you had your bowels open since yesterday?

(Maguire, 1985, pp.1711-1712)

In both the above examples the doctor tries to avoid the central topic of death and the patient's emotion. The doctor in 1) responds to the patient's physical pain ignoring the patient's emotion expressed in the description 'I'm very worried ... ', and the matter of death in 'I'm not going to get better this time'; and in 2) obviously ignores the patient's question 'I'm not going to get out of here, am I?' and again shows his interest only in the patient's physical condition such as his pain and his bowels.

Western doctors seem to be more concerned with disease and science than with their patients and this is what they are taught in medical school, which, as we have seen earlier, emphasizes the 'hard' or physical sciences rather than the social sciences and humanities. Doctors are taught little of how to deal with the patient's anxiety and emotion or how to answer patient's questions, particularly when they are indirect and about the possibility of death, such as 'I'm not going to get out of here, am I?' Death is regarded as a defeat not only for science but also for the doctor, since the doctor has built up his high social standing today through the development of medical science. The existence of those suffering incurable disease and dying violates the doctor's authority and his image of himself as 'a partner of God' (as a scientist) or a healer (Bennet, 1987, pp.81-82). Bennet observes the doctor's typical behaviour in this situation:

> [A]bout death, pain, mutilation, disability and sexuality, he can avoid virtually all real contact with people. This is commonly seen in doctors who never see any patient without assistants of various kinds being present, who always interview their patients across a large desk, who do not willingly halt their forward movement during the ward round, and who certainly never approach closer than the foot of the bed. (Bennet, 1987, p.167)

All these are avoidance strategies, which aim at preventing doctors having to face their own psychological struggle and stress.

With regard to the fear of making mistakes in medical practice, this may be one of the reasons why the doctor tends not to have too close a communication or human relationship with the patient. The doctor is a bearer of good or bad news, and in both cases must face accusations from the patient or the public if he makes a mistake in diagnosis. Thus he may hesitate to state the patient's condition or disease definitely. When the doctor discovers something wrong with his patient, he may not tell the patient about it until her next visit, so that he can examine the matter more in his own mind, because there is always a possibility of error and misdiagnosis. (Lipscomb, 1988, pp.98-99) Hence Western doctors are not always confident in their judgment, and therefore they may not want to answer all of the patient's questions because of the risk of making mistakes. We have seen that the Western doctor has at least two fears relating to medical practice; firstly fear of his patient's death and emotions and secondly of making mistakes, and these fears have led the doctor to defend himself by avoiding any deep communication with the patient. While the public has begun to criticize doctors for paternalism, poor communication, and ignorance of the patient's emotions, we need to consider the doctor's vulnerability when we think of why he has these defensive attitudes towards the patient.

The Doctor's Wound   The doctor's two masks, the mask of the priest/father (symbolic) and the scientist, which interacts in a mysterious way with the doctor's mask of the healer, are accepted more or less both by the doctor and the patient; however, the doctor's vulnerable face as a human being underneath the masks has been ignored by the doctor himself as well as by the patient. Society's over-identification of the doctor with the three masks seems to have made the doctor and the patient forget the fact that the doctor is also a vulnerable person. The healer's mask of the doctor may reinforce the power of the masks of the priest/father and the scientist by integrating the two, but this interaction may not be sufficient to work in an appropriate way for the patient as well as the doctor, unless the doctor understands and cares for his own vulnerability, remembering the idea of the wounded healer. Whether a priest or a scientist, he cannot understand and care for the patient's pain unless he tries to do the same for his own pain. So how the doctor treats his own anxiety, emotion, stress, and depression may be strongly linked with how he treats those of his patients. According to figures published by Her Majesty's Stationary Office, the suicide rate of male doctors in England and Wales from 1970 until 1972 was three times the average for the nation (Registrar General, 1978; cited by Bennet, 1987, p.25). There could be various reasons for this, but the statistics may mean that many doctors do not seem to be good at dealing with their anxiety, stress, and depression, which lead them to commit suicide.

We mentioned earlier under the heading 'Vulnerable Doctors' that modern Western doctors are wounded healers who do not know their own wounds. Indeed, doctors have not been allowed any opportunity in their medical education to stop and think about themselves as vulnerable sentient beings. Nichols, a clinical psychologist, explains that the doctor tends to pay attention to the patient's body thus becoming too objective, particularly when he feels anxious (Nichols, 1984, p.27). This may be because the doctor tries to deny the existence of his anxiety and to get it out of his consciousness. He has established such an unhealthy attitude to his anxiety for a long time since the days of his medical education, when he could be blamed for being emotional under extreme stress and was encouraged to retreat into the objectivity of science and technology. So even if he feels anxiety and stress, he has been required to behave as if feeling nothing. While doctors are not expected to express their stress and anxiety when facing death or shouldering the great responsibility for human life which does not allow for mistakes, they tend to ignore what they are really feeling. Doctors' high suicide rates may then be related to their pain which has not been cared for.

When the doctor understands and cares for his vulnerable human face, he may complete his healer's mask harmonizing it with the other two masks for both himself and his patients, but when he does not do so he may not be able to use the masks in an appropriate way for either himself or his patients. If we accept the traditional view as discussed earlier, that a good healer knows his own vulnerability and therefore can heal others, we can see that the healer's mask is completed the more the doctor appreciates his human vulnerability and the more the other two masks of the priest/father and the scientist are merged into the healer's mask. The doctor's vulnerable face as a human being has been ignored or not seriously considered especially in the modern period as is shown by the high suicide rate, which may show that the doctor cannot be 'a good healer without knowing his own wound'. It is vital therefore to take his vulnerability more seriously so that he can use the mask of the father/priest, and the scientist in an appropriate way for both his patients and himself.

The Hospice Movement and the Doctor-Patient Relationship

As we have seen in the previous two chapters and the early part of this chapter, the time of the Enlightenment was, in relation to the emergence of science, an important transition period for the Western attitude to death and dying, the medicalization of hospitals as distinguished from medieval hospices, and the nature of the doctor-patient relationship. Since this period until the 1960s, the traditional hospice movement lost its power and only survived in a few Christian organizations such as the Sisters of Charity, as through medical science, interest became focused on curing diseases rather than developing hospice-type care. From the 1960s the modern hospice movement, which began in Britain as a strong reaction against the cure-centred dehumanized treatment of patients, has also been a reaction against the way that the doctor's mask of a healer and that of a scientist as well as a father/priest interact. This interaction tends to treat patients merely as objects for clinical treatment and research, pays no respect to patients' rights and autonomy, continues with treatment even in cases of incurable disease, and disregards the doctor's vulnerability. Let us consider now the relationship between the modern hospice movement and the doctor-patient relationship from several points of view.

Purification of the Threefold Guilt

When we discussed the pilgrim-cancer patient metaphor in Chapter 2, we considered that the hospice may 'purify' the threefold guilt of the patient, the family, and the doctor. The doctor has to face the defeat of science and himself as a scientist when he has a lot of difficulty in dealing with the terminally ill and their families because he has not learnt the communication skills or psychological methods for coping with the stress or emotions related to death not only of his patients but also himself. As a result, the doctor may begin to feel guilty about his inability as a scientist or a father/priest, because he conceives his role as giving aggressive treatments to patients whilst ignoring the emotions of patients and their families. In the hospice by contrast, the doctor's role is, first of all, to release patients from pain of different sorts (physical, psychological, spiritual, etc.) rather than to cure their disease, so the doctor does not have to feel guilty but can do something for incurable patients and their families. Likewise, the guilt of cancer patients created by the punitive image of cancer and also the guilt of the family coming from their feeling of uselessness in the face of their loved ones dying in pain, are reduced by the redefinition of the meaning of the disease and of their roles; in other words, cancer patients are identified with 'innocent pilgrims or penitents on the way to salvation' and the family can take part in the patient's dying process because of the informal nature of care in the hospice.

The hospice may be successful in relieving people's guilt, but it does not mean that patients, their families, and carers are relieved from their pain. This pain may involve patients feeling scared of death, being lonely or suffering from some uncontrollable symptoms; their families feeling deep grief over the patients' dying process and bereavement after their death; and carers such as doctors, nurses, and volunteer workers feeling stress and grief in facing death and dying every day. To some extent, therefore, it seems that everyone in hospices is wounded and in pain, but this pain may have an important role in the hospice as we will discuss later.

A Change from the Doctor-Patient Relationship into the Patient-Community Relationship - the Completion of the Healer's Mask

It is understandable that everyone, whether a patient or a carer, will suffer to a certain degree when they are facing death and dying, and this fact is not ignored by hospices, rather all pains and suffering are to be shared within the hospice 'community'. As not only doctors but also many others have important roles in caring for patients, we may not need to think of 'the doctor-patient relationship' as more important than the patient's relationship with other carers. The reason why the doctor-patient relationship has been taken so seriously in Western medical ethics could be that in hospitals the doctor has such power and authority with his scientific knowledge as to be of central importance in decision-making about matters of life and death, which may easily change the patient's destiny. But in hospices the doctor may not be allowed to have this authority in comparison with other carers, because the nature of hospice care is different from that of the hospital, and the patient 'as a pilgrim' is supposed to be at the very centre in the task of completing his pilgrimage through his own will and autonomy, with support from many carers including his family and not from his doctor alone.

So it may be that we need to look at human relationships in hospices in a more holistic way and use the expression 'the patient-community relationship' rather than the doctor-patient relationship. Such community sharing could be considered also from the aspect of the connection between the hospice movement and the Western attitude to death and dying. 'Community sharing' in the matter of death and dying in hospices overlaps with the early Christian attitude to death and dying as explored in Chapter 5, in which the whole community got involved with each person's death and dying, and tried to strengthen the bonds amongst the members of the community on each particular occasion. The hospice philosophy may be reviving the early Christian community sharing of death and dying.

In the notion of 'the patient-community relationship', carers' responsibility is divided more evenly without any concentration on the doctor alone, so their stress can be reduced by sharing it with one another as expressed by Hill:

> The work will inevitably cause pain and bewilderment to some, if not all members of the staff ... Many have to search, often painfully, for some meaning in the most adverse circumstances and yet gain enough freedom from their own anxieties to listen to another's question of distress. (Hill, 1989, p.16)

Carers have to realise that they should not ignore their own needs to share and care for their stress, anxiety, and fear in dealing with patients. This leads us to the idea of 'a wounded healer', in which only those who understand their own vulnerability can heal others. 'A healer's mask' is completed by the recognition and the care of his own pain, but this mask is not only for doctors but also for all the other carers in the hospice team. There is then a more holistic focus on human relationships in hospice care, than emphasizing only the doctor-patient relationship.

The Idea of Vocation

In the pilgrim-cancer patient metaphor in Chapter 2, we saw how cancer patients become pilgrims, and carers act as 'hosts' or 'hostesses' to give 'pilgrims' support on 'their journey' to death so that they can gain 'salvation'. We should not forget, however, that carers are also vulnerable and wounded as we have already seen. As Christ saved sinners by his pain and death on the Cross, carers can help patients in pain by the recognition and care of their own vulnerability. That is to say, they themselves may require a spiritual growth so that they can also take their own 'pilgrimages' together with patients, through finding Christ's pain within both patients and themselves and through supporting patients and sharing their own pains with other carers. We have explored the notion of vocation for doctors as 'priests', but we should now use this concept for all carers, as the idea that only doctors are called to be priest-like as a partner of God or the new 'God' of science may not be significant in the hospice philosophy, where there is no sacred area into which no one except doctors are permitted to enter. The care-centred hospice management may 'ordain' not only doctors from a 'sacred' scientific world as priests but also every carer as 'a wounded healer', because hospice care may be seen as a 'sacred' world in which all those who are involved in caring within it are 'sacred'. This 'sacred' nature may be, however, one of the crucial weaknesses in the paradoxical nature of the pilgrim-cancer patient metaphor as elucidated in the first chapter, because people do not tend to practice the hospice philosophy in their own lives outside of hospice care.

The Healer's Mask and an Individual's Vulnerable Face

As Eliza in Pygmalion says she can be a lady when treated as a lady, and we may be able to fit this idea to the doctor's case by suggesting that the doctor can be 'a good healer' when he is treated as such. What is meant by treating him as 'a good healer' reminds us of the notion of 'a wounded healer'. If society including the doctor himself treats the doctor as a vulnerable human being, the doctor may be able to be a good healer. The reason why the wounded healer can himself heal is that he understands the patient's pain, suffering, and need, from his own experience of them. Vulnerability is, however, an essential part of all sentient beings, and not something external involving a separate role as the word 'mask' implies; in other words, the vulnerable face of a human being is a genuine part of all humans, not of doctors alone. The informal care of the hospice, which does not need specific medical knowledge to the extent that it is needed in cure-centred hospitals, may enable everyone to become a good healer once they understand their vulnerability as humans, and here the healer's mask is very close to the person's vulnerable human face.

Such properties of the healer's mask can be distinguished from that of the doctor in hospitals, where the understanding of his vulnerability may be important and necessary but cannot be enough to do the healer's job because he needs the professional knowledge of medical science and the judgement of how to apply it jointly with the patient's consent. Unlike in hospice-type care, the good healer's mask in hospital-type treatment needs to work together with the mask of the scientist and the father/priest. That means the doctor without special knowledge and skills of medical science cannot be a 'good healer' in hospital-type treatment, even if he understands his vulnerability as a human being. Therefore we may find one of the reasons for the difficulty in applying the hospice philosophy to hospitals lies in the fact that the nature of 'a good healer' is different between hospitals and hospices: in the former the doctor's role is very special and may need to use the mask of a scientist as well as a priest/father with careful awareness of his vulnerable human face, but in the latter the doctor does not take any initiative in the patient's dying process and 'a good healer's face as one of the wounded' can be developed by all the carers, not only the doctor.

The Risk of Destroying the Patient-Community Relationship in the Hospice

While the hospice redefines human relationships within medicine, there is a risk that the doctor will appear in the hospice as a scientist and father/priest once again because terminal care is now becoming more specialised and technical being described as palliative care, in which specific knowledge such as of pain killing drugs is required. The doctor-patient relation may then again become the main relationship which could destroy the hospice-community involvement with the dying process of the patient whilst encouraging a doctor-oriented dying process.

9 Doctors, Patients, and the Japanese Hospice Movement

Introduction

In the same way as we discussed the Western doctor-patient relationship in Chapter 8, we will now analyze the idea of the masks of the Japanese doctor, so that we can understand how the role of the doctor has been defined in Japan. This investigation will be considered together with the Japanese hospice movement in the second section of this chapter. This will help us to discover some of the important characteristics of the Japanese hospice, and to make a comparison with the Western hospice movement in Chapter 10.

The Japanese Doctor-Patient Relationship

The Masks of the Doctor

The Doctor as a Priest In the Middle Ages, to become ill tended to have a religious connotation as it was regarded as a 'kegare' (impurity). In the Japanese classics such as *Genji-monogatari* and *Makura no soshi*, we find a healing activity through prayers and spells, and the person who says the prayers and spells would be considered a priest with a mysterious power to contact the spiritual world and to let evil spirits out from the diseased. We find, for example, a dramatic fight between a priest and a living spirit which had entered into the heroine in the story of *Genji-monogatari* (Mori, 1992, pp.28-29). There also seemed to be the idea of vocation but in a different way from the West. For instance, it was told that Kukai (774-835), in his entrance to the priesthood, was inspired by his mother's dream. It has also been written that many mothers of priests had dreams before their sons' births or in their childhoods, which implied a priesthood for their sons (Armstrong, 1950, pp.13-18). Although these dreams were experienced by mothers, we can still think of the idea of the priesthood as predestined, as it was seen to be related to a natural force or a part of Nature, which may influence an individual to become a priest.

An important point, however, is that the image of those who were called 'doctors' before Japan imported Western science was different from that of priests, because doctors' social status was low while that of priests was considered to be high. Priests seemed to heal the diseased not by skillful surgery but through a mysterious spiritual power to fight against the evil spirits within the sick person's body or to intercede with Nature or God by saying prayers or casting spells. The spiritual power of priests was therefore highly regarded and respected, as priests had the second highest status shared with warriors behind that of the Emperor and feudal lords, but the manual dexterity of doctors was slighted, as we will see when we come to an historical analysis of Japanese doctors' social status. So we need to distinguish the image of priests from doctors in the period before the development of medical science. But the emergence of science in Japan has created the mask of the doctor as a scientist, and this may be seen as 'ordaining' the doctor as 'a priest' because both priests and doctor-scientists heal the apparently incurable by use of a 'mysterious power' (spiritual power for the former and scientific technology or knowledge for the latter). Indeed, scientific technology must have been considered as 'magic' in former centuries.

The Doctor as a Father In this section we consider the doctor as a father.

An honorific title for the doctor The Japanese language requires a change in the way of speaking according to whether the other person is older in age or higher in social status. Japanese people use an honorific title for those older or of higher social status than themselves. Japanese patients always use a term of respect when they speak to the doctor calling him 'Sensei' (a teacher), showing that the patient, whether consciously or unconsciously, acknowledges the superiority of the doctor at the moment of their conversation, and this may encourage the doctor's paternalism. On the other hand, the doctor's way of speaking to his patients is often not honorific but rather imperative, which reinforces the humility of the patient. So their conversation shows clearly a power imbalance between the doctor and the patient, in which the doctor is superior to the patient.

'Omakase' patients Dr Ono proposed the concept of a 'good patient' from the doctor's point of view as follows:

   (i) being obedient to the doctor;
   (ii) respecting the doctor;
   (iii) keeping rules proposed by the doctor;
   (iv) not being assertive;

(v) showing thankfulness to the doctor;
(vi) not doubting the doctor;
(vii) waiting patiently;
(viii) not questioning too much;
(ix) smiling always;
(x) relying completely on the doctor. (Ono, 1979; cited by Yanagida, 1986, p.199; translated by myself.)

Except for (vii) and (ix), these expectations by the doctor of what constitutes a good patient are likely to be those of a father from his children. The doctor may say to the patient: 'You don't have to question it because you are the patient'; 'Don't interfere with the way of my treatment!'; 'Just do what I say to you!' (Anzai *et al.*, 1981, pp.92-93). Physicians have great authority (Yonemoto, 1987, p.218; cited by Ishiwata *et al.*, 1994, p.61) and complete power as patients feel obliged to do what they are told by them (Segawa, 1988, p.170; cited by Ishiwata *et al.*, 1994, p.61). The doctor may feel, therefore, that he is disgraced when the treatment does not go well, and he may become unconsciously punitive towards and blaming of the patient, just as a father is expected to be almighty to his children and may become angry with both himself and his children when he cannot help accepting the fact that he is not perfect.

The patient usually seems to try to be a 'good patient' (i - x) and entrusts the whole process of medical treatment obediently and respectfully to the doctor. Morioka points out that there are many (what he calls) 'Omakase' (the Japanese word for 'entrusting') patients, who say 'I entrust it to you, doctor' when the doctor asks for their views in the medical-decision making process (Morioka, 1989, p.160; cited by Ishiwata *et al.*, 1994, p.61). Some patients even say 'Why must I decide it by myself? Let me leave it with you' (Konishi, 1991, p.465; Takamiya, 1991, p.469). One of the reasons for such a passive attitude of the patient which encourages the doctor's paternalism is that the Japanese tend to want to entrust decisions to another person or to Nature and this has developed in Japanese culture throughout centuries (Morioka, 1989, p.160; cited by Ishiwata *et al.*, 1994, pp.61-2). Another possible reason is that in the long history of feudalism the Japanese mentality has fostered a master-servant relationship, in which an individual readily looks up to those in authority (Kawano, 1988, pp.183-94; cited by Ishiwata *et al.*, 1994, p.62). It is not surprising then that within the doctor-patient relationship, the process of informed consent between physician and patient has not yet been established in Japan. The doctor does not try to wholly share information with his patients nor reveal the true diagnosis, especially in the case of incurable diseases such as advanced cancer (Ishiwata, 1994, p.61). Japanese doctors make all the important decisions themselves and no one criticises or questions their judgments (Becker, 1992, pp.247-48).

The Doctor as a Scientist and Technician

Science has had a strong influence on the modern image of Japanese doctors and in the development of their social status. As with Western doctors, we will look at the history of Japanese doctors' status in this section.

The History of Doctors' Social Status We shall consider this in two parts: from the seventeenth until the mid-nineteenth century, and from the Meiji period to the twentieth century.

From the seventeenth until the mid-nineteenth century In the seventeenth century during the Edo period, doctors were in a low social class together with carpenters and other craftsmen. The Japanese class system in this period was based upon the Chinese one influenced by Confucianism, in which scholars and other intelligentsia (mainly warriors and priests) had the second highest status after the Emperor, the Shogun and feudal lords. The third and fourth classes consisted of farmers and craftsmen, respectively; and the lowest class was that of merchants. In this system, there were those who were called 'Hinin' (not-human), who did not belong to any social class. The doctor was identified with craftsmen in the fourth class since his job was considered as one involving hand skills rather than the intellect, and jobs done by hand were not regarded as requiring intelligence. In this period, not only medicine, but also any other occupation that required special skills and techniques was not regarded as a job for the educated, who should be in a higher class, but as that of the working class. For example, translators were, by definition, given the same high status as warriors, but were in fact looked down on by warriors. An inventor who flew by making a glider was even accused of frightening the public, though he would be called a great scientist today. Scholars in those days had to be theoretical or philosophical rather than practical or scientific. On the other hand, the doctor could succeed economically and was often richer than those in higher classes because his skill was always in demand (Fuse, 1969).

Kaibara Ekiken, a distinguished doctor at that time, taught that the doctor should not seek financial benefit since medicine was 'Jin-jutsu' (the art of love and compassion) which could help the patient through love and compassion. In the name of 'Jin-jutsu', fees were not laid down but depended upon how much the patient could afford. While the job of the doctor was likely to be financially secure, it seemed shameful for the warrior or the educated to be a doctor. When Arai Hakuseki (1657-1725), one of the most distinguished politicians, became unable to make a living for himself and his family, the spirits of the warrior or the scholar in him did not allow him to become a doctor though he was advised to do so. Motoori Norinaga (1730-1801), a Japanese classical scholar, was also a paediatrician and an obstetrician but never left his academic work with the classics, because he felt it impossible for the doctor's work to help him fulfil a man's life. Warriors were considered to be intelligent, high in the social hierarchy, and proud of being so, while becoming a doctor was considered the same as selling the spirit of the warrior in exchange for maintaining one's life and so humbling oneself and losing dignity by doing the dirty manual jobs of medicine. Here, we can clearly see the low status of doctors relating to practical and surgical skills, which were disregarded and even considered to be something shameful to engage in (Fuse, 1969).

From the Meiji period until the twentieth century (1867-1990s) The status of the doctor was becoming higher at the time of arrival of the Meiji Period because, firstly, the concept of intelligence was changed with the introduction of Western science and technology; and secondly, doctors began to take action to improve their social position. The highest seat of learning called 'Shohei-gakusha', which had existed since the Edo period (C17th-C19th) and had provided Confucian education for government officials, was reformed and became the Ministry of Education in 1871. 'Kaiseijo' specialized in the study of the West and introduced foreign languages like English, Dutch, French, and Russian, and Western mathematics for example. Departments of Law, Humanities, and Science were established in Tokyo University, and a Department of Medicine was also opened there in 1877. The government invited Sato Shochu, a great surgeon, to be the head of the department, appointing him 'Dai-Hakase' (great scholar), which was the highest position attainable by a professor in the Meiji period. Although Confucian scholars strongly objected to this appointment of 'great scholar' to a 'mere' school of medicine, which was considered to teach manual-skills which were no more important than carpentry, the government rejected the complaints, emphasizing the importance of introducing Western technologies, and this made a great contribution to raising the status of the medical doctor (Fuse, 1969).

Various medical laws and regulations have become introduced since the 1870s. In 1879, westernized doctors in Tokyo instituted an association to protect their rights and status, and this was an early form of the Japan Medical Association of today, which was legalized by the Home Secretary in that year. With the financial difficulty of hospitals and in line with a proposal by the medical association, the fees for medical treatments were no longer decided by the patient but became fixed by the government. This maintained hospital budgets and led to an improvement in the quality of doctors and moreover guaranteed their rights. As the job of doctors began to be commercialised, they were able to build private hospitals and attract rich patients (Fuse, 1969).

At the beginning of the twentieth century, there was financial panic and a lot of strikes after the Russo-Japanese War and the Japan Socialist Party originating in 1906 was suppressed for articulating 'dangerous thoughts'. However the Japanese trade union movement was born in 1911, and the Japan Communist Party appeared in 1922, and to lessen the strength of the social influence of such bodies, the Japan Medical Association proposed the introduction of health insurance. Finally in 1934 a law relating to National Health Insurance was enacted. The law regarded health care services as merchandise, in which for each medical activity (e.g. medical examination, medication, injection, etc.) fees were paid to the doctor from the government. According to his own personal judgment, the doctor could decide the amount of medication and treatments to give the patient, so the doctor could earn a lot of money the more he administered medical treatments. In spite of this the patient did not have to pay except for a small amount of money relating to his share of the insurance premium, and this is the basis of the system prevailing today (Fuse, 1969).

Since the middle of the nineteenth century, the doctor has increasingly had socio-economic and educational power in Japanese society with the introduction of Western science. This was because science had a strong influence on the development of Japanese medical technology, on the change of image of intellectuals, and on the establishment of the Japan Medical Association, which has improved the doctor's social status. From the 1970s a huge number of private medical and dental universities were established, however, the finance of these private universities is dependent upon the students' entrance contribution and children of doctors have a higher priority to be admitted than others. It is not surprising then that there are many scandals of back-door admissions to medical colleges, since gaining the status of a doctor is almost a synonym for a passport to success in life in terms of economic and social standing (Fuse, 1969).

Having looked at the history of the doctor's status, we find some important points. The first is that the doctor's social standing was low while hand skills were normally not understood as attributes of intellectuals, before the emergence of modern science in Japan. The Japanese doctor was not distinguished from the carpenter and other craftsmen, whose jobs were of manual labour, and so was placed in a lower position in the social hierarchy until Western science arrived in Japan. The second is that the doctor was placed higher socially after the establishment of the medical colleges, in which the surgical and other practical skills of medicine were for the first time highly regarded as intellectual abilities.

Science and Doctors While the Japanese doctor's social status became high along with the emergence of science, some doctors are now interested only in the patient's disease (particularly uncommon or incurable ones) or the process of disease and their symptoms, and make every possible examination regardless of the patient's pain (Anzai, 1981, p.89). In the case of cancer, many patients have acute pains in their terminal stage, but some doctors do not use analgesics which might mask an assessment of the effect of other medical treatments (Oki, 1991, p.33).

Kashiwagi describes how there is a medical doctor ironically nicknamed 'Nat-Kali doctor', who is a specialist in the metabolism of electrolytes, because he is interested only in checking the quantity of natrium (sodium) and kalium (potassium) in the patient's blood and does not go near the bedside of the patient. The interest of this 'Nat-Kali doctor' is to get a scientific result by examining the balance of natrium and kalium in the patient's blood (Kashiwagi, 1991a, pp.92-93). He may think that this will benefit many future patients in the long run, though it gives the current patient unnecessary pain. How much the doctor as a scientist succeeds in curing diseases determines whether or not he can gain a higher position in the medical world. Therefore research on how the doctor helps the patient to die in peace is not attractive to modern Japanese medicine, because death is a defeat of science and of the doctor as a scientist (Nishikawa; cited by Yanagida, 1986, pp.77-78).

Vulnerable Doctors

We are not certain that the Japanese doctor has the same idea of being wounded as his counterpart in the West has, but let us think about the image of a 'wound' in the traditional idea of medicine called 'jin-jutsu', as emphasized by Kaibara Ekiken in the seventeenth century as an important aspect of medical practice. The Chinese character for 'jin' implies 'love and compassion' (Shinjigen, 1964, p.43), and 'jutsu' means 'art'. So in Japan, medicine has traditionally been considered as 'an art of love and compassion'. Compassion in Japanese is 'do-jo', in which the character 'do' means 'same' and 'jo' 'the movement of feelings within the heart' (Shinjigen, *Dictionary of Chinese Characters*, 1964, p.375; translated by myself). So compassion ('do-jo') implies 'to have a movement of feelings within the heart in the same way as the other person'. In the idea of medicine as 'jin-jutsu', doctors are required to treat the patient lovingly and have the same flow of emotions and feelings as the patient has in order to understand his or her pains and heal them. In other words, doctors may need to know about their own pains if they are really to try to feel compassion for patients. If doctors have not had any experience of looking at their own painful emotions such as the stress of frequently experiencing death and dying or the pain of looking at patients in agony or their families in bereavement, they may find it hard to have 'the same flow of emotions' as their patients have in their pain and suffering. Here, we may find the same idea of the wounded healer as described in Chapter 8, who can heal others by his or her wound, or experience and knowledge of pain and suffering. But the doctor's wound or experience of pain and suffering is often repressed and not really recognized by himself, and that means he cannot have the same feeling of pain and suffering as that of his patient. So he does not know how to deal with the patient's pain, apart from treating it merely as a physical pain, which is a matter of science. The doctor's attitude to his emotions and pains will then be reflected in his defensive attitudes towards patients as we will discuss in the next section.

Defensive Attitudes of the Doctor We looked in the earlier section 'The Doctor as a Father', at the fact that Japanese doctors do not want their patients to question or interfere with the method of their treatments. This may come not only from the doctor's over-identification with his own authority but also from his defensive attitude. The doctor often cannot stand silence in his communication with the patient. In the case of the terminally ill, because the doctor has not been educated as to how to deal with the death of the patient, he struggles and does not know what to do or say in front of terminal patients (Mizuguchi, 1991, p.473).

The doctor's fears - fear of the patient's death In the section on the 'Doctor as a Scientist', we talked about the 'Nat-Kali doctor' who was interested only in checking the amounts of Natrium (sodium) and Kalium (potassium) in the patient's blood and did not go near the bedside of the patient. One of the important reasons for his behaviour is his attitude as a scientist as we explored earlier, but another crucial reason could be his fear of the patient's death and emotion related to the person's dying process. The modern Japanese doctor, like his Western counterpart, has learnt in medical school mainly to cure diseases using scientific technologies and has come to regard death as a defeat of medicine and science. The development of medical science has a strong link with the improvement of the doctor's status, as we have previously discussed, so a defeat of medical science might endanger his social standing. Doctors may feel psychologically insecure when they face the reality that they cannot do anything as scientists or priests/fathers who are expected to have the 'mysterious power' of science to heal diseases. So the doctor prefers prolonging the patient's death to accepting his death or letting him die peacefully (Furukawa, 1986, pp.77-78). Thinking that their role is to cure diseases, doctors feel guilty at treating the incurable patient and at his death (Nishimura, 1991, p.92). Moreover, because the Japanese doctor has had little education in dealing with the death of the patient, he does not know what to do or say in front of terminal patients and feels embarrassed when confronted with silence (Mizuguchi, 1991, p.473).

The doctor's fears - fear of making mistakes in medical treatment According to a recent NHK (Japan Broadcasting Corporation) survey, more than 70 percent of doctors themselves regard the doctor as not trustworthy (Becker, 1992, p.250). We need to think about the reason for this from different angles. Firstly, when 70 percent of Japanese doctors consider that doctors in general are not trustworthy, their past or current experiences with other doctors may have led them to this answer. Secondly, there may be cases where they themselves acted unethically or were incompetent in their own medical practice and this made them feel that other doctors were also like themselves. At any rate, this may show that Japanese doctors are not always confident of their abilities and that this lack of confidence could cause them to fear making mistakes. The misuse of the 'mysterious' power of science as a priest/father and scientist is not forgivable because it could harm the patient, sometimes fatally, and this makes doctors fall from the 'sacred' world to that of criminal status, where no longer do the patients or society regard him as 'a holy one'. Moreover, those who are considered to be in such a 'sacred world' as that of doctors and clergy are more readily accused when they commit crimes, than people who are outside such professions.

The Doctor's Wound We are not going to discuss much about the Japanese doctor's wound in its similarity to that of the Western doctor; however, we need to take notice of a feature of it which is unique to the Japanese doctor; that is, the great culture shock which the Japanese doctor feels. In Chapter 6, we explored how death tends to have been something sad for the Japanese rather than frightening because they have accepted it with compassion as a natural event. For Japanese people, death does not seem to have been an enemy but an object of compassion and sadness, and emotion related to the sadness is naturally accepted, because it has been considered to be natural to feel sad about sad things. Japanese doctors, however, are scared of facing the death and dying of the patient and getting involved with the strong emotions of the patient and his or her family.

We analyzed in Chapter 6 how the Japanese might have difficulty in accepting the death of others, but this difficulty is not the same as the doctor's difficulty in accepting his patient's death, because the former is related to their strong identification with the dead, but the latter to the doctor's identification with his role as a scientist and also his ignorance of how to deal with the dying. Sharing emotions and bereavement, and attachment to a dead person's body in the Japanese traditional attitude to death and dying seem to have been an attempt by the people to accept the person's death, but the doctor tends to avoid accepting the patient's death and to be interested in cure-oriented treatment ignoring that the patient is dying. The doctor's attitude does not fit in with what we have discovered about the Japanese attitude to death and dying. It is interesting to consider the transition of the doctor's personality from traditional Japanese to scientific in the process of becoming a doctor since the time of his medical education.   The doctor will experience a big culture shock standing between his Japanese way of perceiving death and dying, and his scientific-oriented way. To change a culture may not be possible or not something that can be done in a hurry, but the Japanese doctor has been almost forced to reject his Japanese attitude to death, which will not be different from other lay Japanese peoples' and which naturally accepts death and emotional issues as they are. The struggle, pressure, and stress, which the doctor must feel in the transition should be taken seriously as a major cause of his wound.

As discussed at the very beginning of this section, there has been a traditional concept in medicine of 'jin-jutsu' (art of love and compassion). Doctors need to know what they are really feeling with their vulnerable human faces underneath the mask of scientist and priest/father, but the society and even the doctors themselves are not aware of their vulnerability as humans, so they may not be able to complete the mask of the 'good healer' carrying out 'jin-jutsu' (art of love and compassion). In other words, the more doctors are aware of and care for their own painful feelings, that is, their own vulnerable faces, the more they can feel compassion for their patients through having 'the same type of feelings and emotions within their hearts'. When doctors and the society care more about this vulnerable face underneath the mask, the doctor may be able to complete his healer's mask. But at present doctors cannot be sensitive and open to the patient's pains of different kinds in relation to death and dying, and instead become very defensive about them, because they tend to ignore their vulnerable faces under the masks.

The Hospice Movement and the Doctor-Patient Relationship

We described in Chapter 3 how with an increasing interest in controlling the pains of terminal cancer patients and in improving the quality of their life, some Japanese doctors began to consider the possibility of hospice care for Japanese patients. But Japanese hospices are expected to develop inside hospitals rather than outside, so the style of the doctor-patient relationship in hospitals may remain to a certain degree also in hospices, because it is not easy for doctors as well as patients to change their attitudes to each other and to the medical process suddenly between hospice care units and the other units, which are often inside the same building or organization. This will be the main issue in our consideration of a connection between the Japanese hospice movement and doctor-patient relationship, and we will discuss it in several aspects in this section.

The first aspect, already discussed in Chapter 3, is that many Japanese physicians, patients, and their families still, to some extent, believe in cure-oriented treatments, which prolong the patient's life even if the person is incurable, so it is possible to imagine that they expect some form of hospital-type cure treatment even in hospice or palliative care units. This means the mask of the doctor as a scientist and father/priest will remain also in hospice care, because 'cure' is more likely to imply scientific methods, which turn doctors into priests through using the 'magical power' of science.

Secondly, doctors often do not tell the true diagnosis to patients, as was shown through an investigation that demonstrated that only 49 percent of patients even in Japanese hospices know their diagnosis and most patients die not knowing the true nature of their disease. Although the importance of telling the truth has begun to be considered in Japan, it is normally not considered as a matter of the patient's right and autonomy but that of the doctor's judgment about whether and how the truth should be told or not (Chapter 3). Therefore, it is the doctor and the family who shoulder all the burden of the 'sin' and 'dirt' of patients even in hospice care. In hospitals, patients may be like children who do not make any decisions by themselves but leave these to the people surrounding them amongst whom the doctor tends to have the greatest authority. But in hospice care wards patients become babies, who are even more passive than children, because they do not know the true diagnosis and are brought to hospice wards often through their families' choice. In this condition, doctors become even more like father-figures.

Thirdly, the problem of the doctor's vulnerability still remains in the hospice, because the aspect of the doctor which will be mainly emphasized is his role as scientist or father/priest, and his vulnerability as a human may be ignored. Doctors may continue to have authority in hospice care, since the traditional doctor-patient relationship will be extended to hospice care units from other units inside the same hospital. Moreover, doctors have traditional authority and nurses are much lower than them in social status and so in the dynamics of their relationship with doctors. The fact that nurses' opinions do not have a strong influence in the Japanese medical culture is, as we have considered in Chapter 3, one of the reasons for the difficulty in developing the hospice movement in Japan. If nurses became equal with doctors in a power balance and both became seen as 'carers', doctors' responsibility for patients would be much reduced and their stress, anxiety, fear, etc. could be more easily shared with others. If doctors' pain is not cared for, at least by themselves, but is repressed, it may be hard for them to feel and accept emotions and feelings within the patient as the expression 'medicine is jin-jutsu' implies. Unless a healer is aware of his vulnerability as a human, the healer's mask is not yet completed in the hospice because the doctor's wound and vulnerability are not cared for as they are not in the hospital. Japanese doctors may find it hard to devote themselves only to the incurable without appropriate psychological support for their vulnerable faces underneath the masks, since it must cause them a lot of psychological as well as physical stress. The way of human relationships in hospice wards, which are inside a hospital organization, may then be carried over from other already existing hospital wards.

The fourth issue is related to that part of the doctor's wound which is unique to Japanese doctors, that is, his culture shock, in which the doctor is forced to change his typical Japanese attitudes to death and dying or emotional issues into the more scientific-oriented ones in the process of becoming a doctor through medical education. In order to fit the hospice ideal into the Japanese people's attitude to death and dying, and to dying cancer patients, who are ordinary Japanese citizens, the doctor may need to revive the traditional Japanese perspective on death and dying as explored in Chapter 6. However, the doctor may still be expected to be a scientist to a certain degree, so he has to keep a balance between his traditional perspective and the scientific approach to death and disease in order to overcome the culture shock. There is then a complicated situation in which Japanese patients are expected to have the traditional Japanese perception of death and dying, so they want to die in the way which suits this perception, however, at the same time, they expect the doctor to perform curative treatment to some degree even if they are dying, which may be opposed to their Japanese ideal of death. The reasons for this complex and paradoxical reaction of patients might be that they do not know the nature of their disease as incurable and also do not have a strong awareness of their own individual rights or know exactly what they want doctors to do for them, because they act as 'babies' obedient to their 'fathers'. Modern Japanese patients seem to accept their fate of death together with the nature of the dying process by entrusting it to their doctors.

As we have considered already, it is difficult for Japanese hospices to create a new philosophy of treating patients differently from hospitals' ways because hospices tend to be established inside hospitals; in other words, it is not realistic to imagine that one hospital ward called a 'hospice' or a 'palliative care' unit can develop as a reaction against what is going on in other units inside the same building. So Japanese hospices may mirror the hospital's way of viewing the doctor-patient relationship. However, there might also be a slight possibility that the unique existence of hospice care units itself could have an influence on the way of treating patients in other hospital units, if Japan clarifies and realizes the concept of hospice care through building up a philosophy suitable to its culture, and succeeds in creating an interactive relationship between hospice and hospital wards inside one building.

10 Doctor-Patient Relationships and the Hospice Movement

A Comparison of Doctor-Patient Relationships in the West and in Japan

Similarities

Important similarities underlie the fact that modern medicine has been dependent upon science, which has changed the concept of medicine, the doctor's status and his roles. Medical students are educated to become 'scientists', who attempt to conquer diseases and death, and are not allowed to be emotional in their anxieties and stress since this may disturb them when they are expected to be objective in their medical training and practice. Obtaining a massive amount of knowledge in medical science, they become doctors who can use the 'magical power of science in order to cure diseases'. There is, however, a limit to which the doctor with the mask of scientist and priest/father is supposed to have magical power, since he may sometimes have to face the reality that he cannot cure some patients who are fatally ill, such as advanced cancer patients. He has learnt to deal with diseases scientifically or objectively but has not had enough knowledge and training to develop good communication with the dying and their families or to deal with any emotional problems they have. Death is considered to be the defeat of science and of the doctor as a scientist, so it does not seem to be easy for the doctor to accept it.

In relation to the doctor's denial of death and emotions relating to it, the doctor's defensive attitude before their patients is also similar between the West and Japan. The doctor tends to speak or question more than the patient does, and sometimes does not even allow the patient to interfere with his medical practice. Doctors also avoid any painful issues like death whether consciously or unconsciously by changing the topic or showing interest only in the physical symptoms of the patient or adopting a distant attitude toward the patient.

Both the Western and Japanese doctors seem to wear the mask of scientist and priest/father, and the masks have a great power and authority in their interaction with their healer's mask; in other words, because they

147

are healers, the two masks have power in their relationship with patients, and as we explained earlier not everyone with scientific skills can have the same authority and power as the doctor (Chapter 4). The power and authority having emerged from the interaction between the mask of scientist/priest/father and that of healer may sometimes work in a harmful way for the patients, for example, it could violate the patient's autonomy and rights. On the other hand, the patient seems to expect the doctor to have the power if it works in an appropriate way for the patient. The problem is that there may be a conflict between the patient's expectation towards the doctor's masks and the way in which the doctor actually uses them. One of the reasons for the conflict could be considered from the aspect of the doctor's 'vulnerable face' as a human being underneath the masks, because the conflict may be, in part, related to the lack of understanding of the doctor's vulnerability. The doctor's defensive or aggressive attitude to the patient sometimes may originate from the doctor's fear of death, of making mistakes, and accepting his incapacity in dealing with the terminally ill. Doctors have not been taught how to deal with their emotions, anxiety, stress, etc. during or after their medical education. As the idea of the wounded healer in the West or of medicine as 'jin-jutsu' (an art of love and compassion) implies, doctors may not be able to complete their healer's mask unless they understand and care for their own wound and vulnerability so that they can understand patients' pain or feel compassion (Do-jo: the same flow of emotions) for it.

The West and Japan are strikingly similar in terms of the doctor's scientist/priest/father mask in the interaction with his healer's mask, and in the matter of his uncompleted healer's mask due to ignorance of the doctor's vulnerable face as a human underneath the masks.

Differences

The Doctor's Masks We will discuss these under the headings: a father figure, and a scientist.

A father figure We discussed in the first section on 'Similarities' that the West and Japan are similar concerning the doctor's role in relation to the idea of masks, but now need to recognise also the differences between them from the cultural aspect of human relationships. Firstly let us think about the doctor as father figure in the West and Japan. There is the image of the doctor as 'a teacher' both in the West and Japan, and this relates to the doctor's paternalism in the two, as the English word 'doctor' comes from the Latin 'docere' which means 'to teach' and the Japanese doctor is normally called 'sensei' which means 'a teacher'. If there is the idea that patients are like students obedient to their doctors as teachers, we find this both in the West and Japan. As Japanese patients often say to their doctors 'I entrust you with it', it may be imagined that Western patients say something similar, which implies the doctor's superiority to the patient in medical decision-making. This is because, whether in the West or Japan, doctors tend to speak and question more than patients do, and doctors are those in 'a sacred world' of science, which not everyone can glimpse or explore.

Such a similarity may, however, have a different meaning and implication at a deep level between the two, since the Western doctor's paternalism may be unique in the individualistic Western world, where the individual's right to decision-making is normally taken for granted, while Japanese society is not likely to take special notice of individual decision-making even outside the medical field. In other words, the doctor's paternalism exists in Japan as a reflection of ordinary life, and this must be distinguished from the Western doctor's paternalism in an individualistic society, where individual rights and respect for autonomy are part of ordinary life. Therefore Japanese people may say 'I entrust it to you' not only in the doctor-patient relationship but also in different relationships taking place in their community. This is because, as we have explained earlier in this chapter and in former chapters, it has been common in Japanese society throughout the centuries that important decisions for an individual's life are made by or with those around him. This may be seen in the fact that Japanese doctors normally do not tell the true diagnosis to the patient but to the patient's family if the patient has got an incurable disease, and that the doctors have the authority to make a judgment about whether or not the diagnosis should be told to the patient. It is difficult for Japanese people to pay attention to the doctor's paternalism as a problem in these social circumstances. The doctor's paternalism or his ignorance of the patient's rights and autonomy is considered to be a problem only in societies like the Western countries, where ordinary people are more strongly aware of individual rights than the Japanese lay public are. To change the doctor-patient relationship into a non-paternalistic one in Western societies would merely be to apply the ideas of rights, self-determination, autonomy, etc., which have been taken seriously already as a set of basic values in ordinary day-to-day life, but on the other hand, in Japan this would mean to change the culture as a whole.

A scientist We have described how the doctor's role as scientist is similar between the West and Japan, and has changed the concept of medicine, the doctor's status, and the doctor-patient relationship. But how the mask of the scientist for doctors is made in Western medicine seems to differ from Japanese medicine. As we have seen in the history of the doctor's status (Chapters 8 and 9), in the West science has developed over at least two hundred years since the Enlightenment in the eighteenth century while in Japan it has been introduced within a century by absorbing Western science. Accordingly, Western medical science has been cultivated gradually in the West but suddenly in Japan. Western people may have proceeded from one step to another in the long process of the development of science accepting it or sceptical of it, whether the adjustment is successful or not. Japanese people started from the middle of the stairway not from the bottom, because they imported Western science, when it had already achieved a degree of development, so the Japanese mind has not been given enough time to cope with or make philosophical enquiry into the scientific approach to medical practice. The Enlightenment bore medical science but at the same time made a 'safety net' from the enquiring mind of analytical philosophy, which approaches the world by a particular form of reasoning, so that the net can catch Western medicine's problems through the emergence of a science that is 'walking a tightrope'. But Japanese medical science has developed without simultaneously creating such 'a safety net'.

The Doctor's Vulnerable Face There is a resemblance between the West and Japan in the fact that the doctor's fear of death and of making mistakes constantly puts pressure on him, and that this pressure is reflected in his defensive or aggressive attitude to his patients. So, the doctor is vulnerable in the West as well as in Japan but his vulnerable face under the masks tends to be ignored by society and even by himself. His wounds, which could come from stress, anxiety, fear, or pressure, are therefore in part the cause of the doctor's paternalism, surface communication, and ignorance of the patient's emotions. But in the case of Japanese doctors, as discussed in Chapter 9, they have an extra difficulty which Western doctors do not have, because they suffer from the dilemma between their traditional attitude to death and dying, and their scientific way of dealing with them. We have seen that the Japanese attitude to death and dying has not significantly changed throughout centuries, and that it is likely that Japanese people will accept death as a fate, to be treated with sadness. Japanese doctors stand in a difficult position, in which they may feel obliged to achieve their tasks as 'scientists' while at the same time they sympathise with the traditional way their patients and the patients' family look at death, in which death is something sad and something to be resigned to. On the other hand, the Western attitude to death and dying has changed at a deep level involving the moral value of people, particularly after the beginning of de-Christianization, so not only doctors but also lay people in the modern Western world generally may feel death as a defeat of human potentiality. In this sense, the Western doctor does not have the dilemma which the Japanese doctor has.

The Doctor-Patient Relationship in Relation to the Hospice Movement in a Comparison between the West and Japan

The Patient-Community Relationship

We have made a comparison between the Western and the Japanese doctor-patient relationships and now will discuss the contrast in connection with the hospice movement. The Western hospice movement has developed as a reaction to the cure-centred dehumanized treatment of patients and also the mode of human relationships in the care of the dying in hospital, where the doctor-patient relationship is very much central. In the Western hospice, everyone can be 'a healer' because of the informal nature of treatment, which is not likely to require specific medical knowledge apart from the use of drugs for pain control. We may not need then to consider the patient's relationship with the doctor as more important than the relationship with other carers. It may be possible to think about human relationships as a whole in the Western hospice, which often has its own building isolated from hospitals and has developed as a strong reaction to the modern hospitalization of the terminally ill. In the case of the Japanese hospice, however, the notion of the patient-community relationship may not be applicable, because Japanese hospices tend to be expected to develop within hospitals, which are very much doctor-oriented. It is not easy for Japanese hospices to create a new philosophy of treating patients in different ways when they are inside the doctor-centred hospitals, so it is more likely that human relationships inside hospices mirror the hospital's; in other words, the doctor may continue to wear the mask of scientist and priest/father in the hospice, which educes a great authority in interaction with his healer's mask.

   In the Japanese hospice, because of the difficulty in establishing the patient-community relationship and the tendency to keep the doctor-patient relationship as the centre of human relationships, the doctor's responsibility for the patient in this medical process is still emphasized or even strengthened in the case of incurable cancer patients in regard to his non-disclosure of the true diagnosis. While the Western hospice movement has widened the doctor-patient relationship, compared with that which takes place in hospital, developing more as a human relationship at a community level, the Japanese hospice may continue with the hospital approach to doctor-centred human relationships.

The Doctor's Vulnerability

As to the doctor's vulnerability, the Western hospice 'community' does not tend to concentrate responsibility for the patient only on the doctor, but shares it amongst all the carers including the doctor and the patient's family. This may reduce the doctor's stress, compared to his practice in the hospital. Also, carers' emotions, stress, anxiety, etc. are shared at a community level. Applying the idea of the wounded healer explored in Chapter 8, such care and sharing of emotions and vulnerability in the hospice community could help the doctor to complete the 'healer's mask' if one can really heal others through one's wound and understanding of one's own vulnerability. The healer is, however, not only the doctor, but everyone else taking part in the informal nature of hospice care. So the whole community of the hospice attempts to complete the healer's mask by sharing the vulnerability through a deep understanding.

On the other hand, the Japanese doctor's pain may remain not cared for even in hospice care, because the responsibilities of treating patients are still too much on the doctor's shoulders, where the traditional doctor-patient relationship is extended from hospital care to the hospice care unit. In the same way that the doctor's stress and anxiety are treated in hospital care, they are also likely to be treated in hospice care since the hospice or palliative care unit tends to be inside the hospital building or institution. So 'the community sharing' of carers' vulnerability, which includes the doctor's vulnerability, does not readily occur in the Japanese hospice. Only doctors are entitled to wear the 'mask of a healer', but the healer's mask has not yet been completed due to their and the society's ignorance of doctors' own vulnerability, which may make them find it hard to feel compassion for and understand the pain and suffering or vulnerability of their patients.

An interesting point is, however, that the Western hospice's community sharing of carers' vulnerability may be limited within the hospice building or the hospice institution or where the hospice care is taking place. We have seen in Chapter 2 on the hospice movement in the West that there is a paradoxical difference between the public attitude to the hospice movement and to death and dying outside hospice care, as the analogy of the greenhouse and strawberries shows. People are keen on building a lot of greenhouses (hospices) so that they can taste strawberries (the hospice type care and sharing of death, dying, and related emotional issues) in the wasteland (outside hospice care), but do not try to grow strawberries in their own garden so it remains a wasteland, where no strawberries grow. The existence of the hospice is in a way evidence that people cannot grow strawberries in their own garden, and reinforces the conditions outside the hospice. Likewise, the community sharing of the vulnerability of carers might be very much dependent upon the hospice organization, because in the outside world, whether in hospital or in people's ordinary life, its philosophy has not spread throughout Western society, where death and emotional issues are not openly discussed, and the human vulnerability of people in a caring position such as doctors is not taken seriously. On the other hand, the Japanese situation is the other way round in this regard, because except within medicine, the community sharing of death and emotional issues is still a strong tradition in contemporary Japanese society.

11 Conclusion

In this chapter, the final part of the book, we, first of all, need to clarify what is the meaning and the value of our cultural comparison of the hospice movement between the West and Japan. Although we have limited the range of our discussion to the issues around the hospice movement, we have seen that the topic involves cross-cultural matters such as the form of human relationships, perspectives on death, and awareness of the self.

In regard to Japanese medicine, it is right to say, as we have discussed in the former three chapters, that Japanese doctors have been suffering from a dilemma between their traditional Japanese attitude to death and dying and their scientific attitude, and that certain concepts from modern Western medical ethics and the hospice movement, such as 'truth telling' may not easily suit the Japanese. At the same time it does not seem right to say that there is such a thing as 'perfect' cultural relativism which means that different cultures are unable to share moral values and in which ethical issues become merely a matter of culture. For instance, medical science, which has dramatically changed the nature of Western medicine, might be new to the Japanese mind, but on the other hand, the basic principles of the scientific approach to diseases such as the cause-effect relationship are not a completely new idea for Japanese people. There had long been such an attitude to events in the world by which people attempted to understand various phenomena in terms of a cause-effect relationship. For example, there was a man who made a glider in the Edo period and the invention would have been impossible without his understanding of cause-effect principles (see Chapter 4). So, while Western science was imported by the Japanese people, its basic interpretation of events in the world was not totally strange to them. This may be one of the reasons for the fact that Japanese medicine and culture have succeeded in part, in applying imported Western medical science and technology to Japanese medicine.

We have taken cultural differences seriously throughout this book, but it is not because, as we have already emphasized in the introduction to this study, we would like to use our investigation for the purpose of finding a clear cultural borderline between the West and Japan. If we regarded Japanese culture or Japanese medicine as completely different from Western culture or medicine, and wanted to consider Japanese medicine completely independently from Western influence, we must immediately throw away Western medical science which has made a tremendous contribution to curing various diseases in Japanese patients. This is unlikely to happen in today's science-oriented Japanese medicine, and it is right that Japan should continue to enjoy benefits from it. As Japanese medicine has developed under Western influence since the end of the last century, it cannot suddenly close the door to the West and cultivate a 'pure Japanese medicine', and that means we will have to consider the future of Japanese medicine together with Western medicine. The question of whether or not such a relationship between Western and Japanese medicine is successful depends upon how we look at the difficulties in applying the methods of the former to the latter. Therefore, it is not that the hospice movement and its Western cultural values can never be relevant to Japanese culture and that they can be entirely cut off from one another. Nevertheless, we should still accept that there are some significant differences and difficulties, which make it hard for Japan to bring the Western hospice philosophy into Japanese medical culture. In this study, we have attempted to illuminate what they are in order to discover some crucial questions when considering how the idea of the Western hospice might be brought to Japan; in other words, this clarification of the problems is our primary interest in this work. So, as mentioned in the beginning of this book, we will not attempt to give any straightforward answers to the questions, but will now try to find some clues to solving them in this concluding chapter.

A 'Japanese Pilgrimage' Not Begun - the Japanese Hospice as a Myth

One of the most significant difficulties in importing the Western hospice movement into Japanese medicine is the fact that Japanese terminally ill patients cannot be 'pilgrims', because this notion is deeply related to the underlying philosophy of the Western hospice, as we have shown in Chapter 2. The reason for this 'pilgrimage which has not begun' is that the Japanese people have a different perspective concerning 'self', pain, diseases, and death from that of Western people.

Japanese terminal cancer patients are not the same as Western patients. 'Cancer pilgrims' in the West know what their 'crosses' are (dying of cancer pain, which involves both a physical as well as a psychological experience), and they take responsibility for their crosses of pain and suffering. They make important medical decisions on their own. In this active way of approaching their pain and death, the disclosure of the true nature of the disease, as an incurable cancer, is essential. While Western medical science has attempted to conquer the fear of death by denying death itself in its cure-centred approach towards diseases, Western hospices may be now trying to confront the fear of death by making an effort to control pain, giving the dying psychological and spiritual support, and so changing the meaning of death from a frightening thing, which should not be talked about, into the gate to salvation waiting for the patient at the end of his or her 'pilgrimage'.

An interesting point here is that, whether through science or the hospice (both in medieval and modern times), the West seems to have actively challenged 'death', so as to overcome the fear of death. Medical science has attempted to overcome the fear by denying death itself in its tremendous effort to cure diseases and to prolong the average life-span, and on the other hand, the hospice has done it by facing and accepting death actively through the idea of 'taking a pilgrimage whilst carrying a cross'. The two approaches to death are different from one another, but are similar in the matter that both are trying to actively fight against the fear of death in their own ways.

Indeed, Western people began their pilgrimages from the twelfth century partly because of their fear of death, when they began to be more aware of their individual selves. This rise of individualism is deeply connected with the Western fear of death, since the consciousness of one's own self makes a person aware of his own death, which he has to deal with on his own. Before the beginning of the de-Christianization of Europe from the eighteenth century, people in the West tried to overcome their fear of death through their religious faith in God and the resurrection, as expressed in their pilgrimages, and since then they have tried to deny death itself through the perception of the role of science and technology, which have led to the cure of many diseases. But now, both ways of overcoming the fear of death are becoming irrelevant, because whilst people have lost their faith in God, medical science is having to admit its limitations in conquering death by curing the incurable. Not only has science failed to cure some diseases like advanced cancer but also it has increased the pain and fear of the dying process by its aggressive treatment.

To some extent the hospice movement has emerged in the West, in order to deal with this fear together with the physical as well as psychological pain, by redefining the care of the dying.

The Japanese people have not had such a long history of the 'fear of death' and of conquering it, but have traditionally tended to accept death and disease in a relatively passive way. There might be of course some cases in which the Japanese were not just passive towards death, for example, Japanese warriors committed 'harakiri' suicide (by cutting open the abdomen) in cases where they lost their battles. This was considered to be an active attitude to death, and was done as an active acceptance of their death and destiny with dignity and courage. We may find some similarity between the spirit of these warriors and the idea of the Western 'hospice pilgrims' in their active acceptance of death, as we can see that the former committed suicide to die with dignity and the latter took their own 'crosses' of pain to overcome the fear of death, while both in their own ways accepted their destiny.

A vital difference between the two, however, is that the Japanese warriors are unlike the Western 'pilgrims', since the destiny of the Japanese warriors depended upon that of their Lords and associated groups in the feudal system. The warriors were not allowed to decide the matter of their own life and death by themselves. 'Harakiri-suicide' was what they had been taught to do for the purpose of avoiding a shameful death, which dishonoured their social groups and Lords, rather than to gain salvation or eternal life by conquering death as in the Christian belief. This strong awareness of their group responsibilities for the community and their Lords rather than the awareness of themselves as individuals does not therefore match the idea of the 'Western hospice pilgrimage', which requires one to die his or her own death as an individual by shouldering his or her own 'cross' of pain and has a different meaning for each individual's life. The Japanese mentality has not had a strong consciousness of individuality in its history, because the group or the community has been considered to be more important than each individual. Without an emphasis on 'self-awareness', the idea of the hospice 'pilgrimage' is impossible, and this is why the Japanese who do not have this strong self-awareness cannot be 'pilgrims'.

Japanese terminal cancer patients are more like 'babies'. Apart from the Japanese passive acceptance of death and disease, and their group orientation, which we have already described, another crucial reason for this 'babyness' is that they do not or are often not allowed to (even if they may want to) take individual responsibility for their disease, because the true nature of the disease is often not told to them. The question of telling the diagnosis in the case of incurable diseases reflects how much patients can or are forced to take responsibility for their disease and death, and also how the meaning of each of their existences is defined in the culture. At the point the diagnosis is told to the patient, he can more or less control the situation by his own medical decision, and can consider what sort of attitude he is going to take towards his disease, pain, death, people around him and the rest of his life. This is necessary for him to take his own 'pilgrimage' shouldering his 'cross' of pain.

But if the diagnosis is concealed, the patient is not in control of the situation and his family and carers have to decide what would be the best for him, and at this stage the meaning of the rest of his life is almost totally defined by those around him. In Japanese hospice care, half of terminally ill cancer patients still do not know their diagnosis, and this is partly because Japanese hospices are being developed inside hospitals. This is claimed to be for economic reasons but also means that Japanese hospice care is likely to be similar in nature to hospital type treatment of patients, in which a diagnosis of incurable disease is normally hidden from them. Japanese incurable cancer patients are 'sent to' hospice wards often without knowing the name of their disease and their destiny of death (apart from if they sense it by intuition), and so cannot make any medical decisions but rely on others to do so on their behalf. This is very far from the idea of a 'pilgrim' in the Western hospice movement.

While the Western and the Japanese hospice movements are similar in their primary interest in pain-control of terminal cancer, Japanese hospice care does not have some of the other important features of the Western hospice movement, which are firstly its active approach to death and pain shown by the idea of pilgrimage and 'taking up one's own cross', and secondly an individual responsibility for the matter of disease and death in relation to the disclosure of cancer diagnosis. These two vital features of the Western hospice philosophy have not been applied to the current Japanese hospices, though the Japanese seem to believe that they have imported or are going to bring the Western hospice concept to their country.

We may now, therefore, need to question whether the Japanese hospice can be called a 'hospice', and whether 'the Japanese hospice as a borrowed Western invention' is a mere 'mythology'. The Japanese image of a 'hospice' seems to be of a place, (a) where you can let your loved one die in peace with as little as possible physical and psychological pain surrounded by kind carers and the family, and (b) where you do not have to let your loved one know the sad news about matters like death which entail the pressure of individual responsibility for disease and death. Now (a) can be shared with the Western hospice ideal, but (b) may not be able to coexist with the idea of the Western 'pilgrimage' involving a 'cross', a strong awareness of the individual self, and the attempt to actively accept and overcome the fear of death. In taking the hospice philosophy from the West, Japan has transfigured it so as to suit its own culture, but in this 'transfiguration' of the hospice concept the Japanese hospice may no longer be appropriately called a 'hospice' any more.

Is the Japanese Hospice Really a Hospice?

Telling the Diagnosis

If Japan wants to call its developments in terminal care 'hospice care' by denying the possibility of 'the hospice as a myth' and by regarding them as 'real', the first thing that must be done is to tell the patient about the fact that he has got an incurable cancer, because this is deeply related to how the hospice philosophy (in the West) defines the meaning of the patient's life and death during his dying process. In the Western hospice concept, the patient is supposed to take responsibility for his life and death as an individual, so that he can define the meaning of the rest of his life and how he will spend his dying process in his preparation for death. It is impossible for the patient to do this without knowing his situation in which he has got an incurable disease and is going to die. Now, if Japan tried to spread 'truth telling' throughout the country, the situation would be very different from that in the West. This is because Japanese culture has not really encouraged the individual to have a strong awareness of self and to determine the matter of his life and death on his own, and this means that the Japanese people have not had a strong awareness of individual responsibility for their lives. Letting a person take responsibility for his own disease, and life and death seems to be something which Japanese individuals have not done in past years. Telling the diagnosis in the case of incurable disease may imply something more than just 'telling' and implies 'changing' the Japanese patient's way of living suddenly at the very end of his life as compared with his past years.

We have suggested throughout this book that there is a degree of infantilization of incurable cancer patients both in Western and Japanese hospices. In the former the hospice provides patients with a certain ideal way of dying as a process of 'pilgrimage', and in the latter patients die without knowing the nature of their disease and with people around them making all the judgments about what their best interests would be during their dying process. The implication of this infantilization, however, needs to be distinguished in each case, because Western 'cancer pilgrims' are not allowed to die as 'babies', and Japanese 'cancer babies' cannot be like 'pilgrims'. The Western way of infantilization may not be possible in the Japanese hospice, nor the Japanese way in the Western hospice. If Japan attempts to develop 'a real hospice', it will have to allow for the telling of the diagnosis to incurable patients who are not in a position to be like Western cancer 'pilgrims' but will respond as 'babies'. Whether as 'pilgrims' or 'babies', it must be difficult for any person to learn that he or she has got an incurable cancer and is going to die in the near future, and such persons need physical and psychological support. But it would seem likely that the 'babies' may need far more support or a different form of support than the 'deserted sinners', if they are to be transformed from 'babies' to 'pilgrims', who become individual responsible adults, in order to make the Western way of infantilization possible for the Japanese hospice.

Also it must be remembered that the Japanese people have difficulty in accepting others' deaths rather than their own death. This could be a hidden and subconscious reason for concealing the diagnosis in Japan. It is too extreme a position to say that the Japanese people have had no fear of death, but it is also true that, in comparison with Western culture, the Japanese have tended to accept death in a rather passive way as a natural order of the universe. We might then wonder what problems would be caused by the disclosure of an incurable cancer diagnosis to the family rather than the patient. The family will have to bear a great burden of responsibility in telling their loved one that she is going to die and hearing themselves announcing 'the death penalty' to her. While they may feel guilty in lying to their loved one, 'not telling the truth' may have its own benefit for them since they can continue to treat their loved one as though she was not dying and not suffering from any incurable disease. While Japanese cancer 'babies' need even more support than Western 'pilgrims' in the case of the disclosure of the diagnosis, we also have to consider that their families may need more support than Western families.

The Transition from a Sad Death to a Frightening Death

The West has, as we have already mentioned, had a long history of actively controlling and changing events in the world rather than passively accepting them. In the awareness of death as an event affecting individuals in the period from the twelfth century until the eighteenth century, people took pilgrimages for their salvation so that they could overcome the fear of death by their faith in heaven, resurrection, and everlasting life. Since the Enlightenment, and the emergence of science, they have tried to overcome the fear of death by denying death itself through focusing on curing diseases. There seems to have been a determination to conquer the fear of death in Western history, but Japan has not made any special effort to confront this fear because there has not been a strong consciousness of the fear itself. Through the idea of a 'sad death', the Japanese people throw themselves into the cycle of Nature with a perception of their existence as a part of Nature. This involves compassion for themselves and all other creatures, which are seen as frail and impermanent by their nature.

If it were possible for Japanese patients to become 'pilgrims' in hospice care, this would mean strengthening their awareness of their lives as individuals, who have their own purpose and meaning, which is not necessarily the same as that of their community. Ironically, this would entail the beginning of the perception of death as something to be feared in Japan, because an individual awareness of one's life will also increase that of death. Death will, then, become more like an object of fear than that of traditional sadness.

Suggestions for the Japanese 'Hospice'

Should Japan Change?

The question to be considered here is whether the Japanese should change their cultural values in the direction of Western values. The fear of death is one of the problems which the West has had for a long time, and there is no sense in which Japan would want to import that fear. We are also not sure if it is better that Japanese patients become more independent through becoming 'pilgrims' so that they 'take up their crosses on their pilgrimage' but remain infantilized in the way of the Western hospice. It is not ideal to import the Western hospice with its hidden problems whereby those who are dying or in bereavement or diagnosed as having an incurable disease become 'strangers' like 'pilgrims' in their own society, and people become unable to talk about emotional issues and the matter of death outside hospice care. Unless Japanese cancer 'babies' become 'pilgrims', they do not have to be regarded as 'strangers' and death does not have to be the object of strong fear for Japanese people as it is for Western people, but once the hospice becomes a 'reality' (not a myth any more), this may happen because the problems underlying the modern Western hospice movement will also become a 'reality'. So we should question now whether Japan really needs to bring unreconstructed hospices to its country.

There is a good case to be made that the Japanese perspective on death should not be changed from that of a 'sad death' into a 'frightening death'; and that Japanese cancer patients should not become 'pilgrims' in modern society. Also 'greenhouses' or isolated hospices should not be created, because their existence provides evidence of conditions outside hospice care which are 'too cold' to grow 'strawberries' (the hospice ideal of the care of the dying) and so reinforces 'the coldness'. Throughout the centuries, the Japanese people have shared the event of death and dying without building hospices and without any strong fear because of their passive attitude to the matter and their lack of awareness of themselves as individuals in a group-oriented society. There would seem no good reason for destroying this cultural tendency, which is not likely to be harmful but can be a strong advantage for the Japanese people.

Can Japan Change and, If So, What Should Be Changed?

Japan does not have to abandon its culture in relation to its attitude to death and dying, because it has helped its people to accept and share the matter of death without their being a strong fear of death. So this non-individualistic society with its passive attitude towards death, does not need to import the 'Western fear and isolation'. On the other hand, this does not mean that the current way of caring for the dying in Japan, particularly for terminal cancer patients, does not need to change or be improved. There are various problems caused mainly by medical science's perspective on humans and the corresponding doctor-patient relationship, which have brought a lot of physical as well as psychological pain to Japanese patients, their families, and their carers.

Some aspects of Western hospice methods such as the physical as well as psychological symptom control of terminal cancer have much to offer Japanese patients, though cocaine is not legally permitted in Japan. In fact, Japan seems to have tried to import the ideas of the Western hospice movement mainly out of their interest in pain control of incurable cancer patients. So, it may be necessary for Japan to use some of the Western hospice methods for the care of terminal cancer patients more or less directly, without completely rejecting the way of the Western hospice. Modern Japanese medicine has been deeply influenced by Western medical science and therefore it is not realistic to think about the future of Japanese medicine in total isolation from Western influence.

The Possibility of Disclosing a Diagnosis of Incurable Cancer Concerning the issue of terminal cancer patients' pain, we have to remember again the different attitudes to pain and suffering between Western cancer 'pilgrims' and Japanese cancer 'babies'. The main difference is the matter of whether the person has an active or a passive attitude to pain and suffering. Remembering the Passion of Jesus in the New Testament, he had to accept the destiny of death but at the same time had to actively walk towards it by shouldering his cross. The Western hospice may be understood by analogy with those who in some way supported Jesus before he reached his destiny: firstly the angel who encouraged and consoled him in the agony of Gethsemane while he had difficulty in accepting what was going to happen to him afterwards; secondly, the Cyrenian called Simon who carried the cross on behalf of Jesus because Jesus was becoming so frail; and finally the woman called Veronica who wiped his face. All this help was in fact to assist Jesus in going on to Calvary to be crucified. This is support to someone who tries to actively achieve his purpose or accept his destiny, but Jesus may not have had this support if he had not walked continuously towards Calvary. Using this analogy for the Western hospice patient, he should receive appropriate pain control by a team of carers, but he himself has to take some part in this process, by knowing his diagnosis and making his own decisions about the matter of life and death.

Such a 'road to Calvary' is not realistic for the Japanese cancer 'babies' since they and their crosses have to be carried on carers' shoulders while they are 'sleeping'. Even in psychological care like that of the 'angel' who consoled Jesus, it is difficult for the 'angels' of hospice care to console the Japanese cancer baby who does not know his destiny but is crying in pain without knowing the cause of the pain. For example, Client-Centred Therapy, one of the most common counselling methods in Japan, which was introduced by the American psychologist Carl R Rogers, is not easily applicable to the Japanese terminal patient. The first reason is that this form of approach to the patient is impossible without the counsellor being honest with himself and the client. The core of the problem here is again related to the matter of 'truth telling'. As long as the diagnosis is not told to the patient, the 'angel', 'Cyrenian', and 'Veronica' cannot take part in Japanese hospice care. As long as the mainstream policy of Japanese medicine is not to disclose the incurable cancer diagnosis, it is inevitable that pain control is given to the patient without his being involved in the decision-making process and the doctor's paternalism continues to be strong in Japanese medicine, whether in hospitals or hospices.

Hoshino, one of the pioneers of modern Japanese bioethics suggests that the diagnosis should be revealed after studying a suitable way of telling for each patient, and the patient's 'right *not* to know' should also be respected (Hoshino, 1991, pp.104-12). But in order to find 'a suitable way' for the patient, the doctor needs to know not only the patient's physical condition but also his or her mental condition, personality and temperament. But it is not easy even for trained psychologists to analyze the personality of an individual, and it is doubtful that the doctor who has no psychological education can achieve this task. A danger is that the patient cannot take part in this search for 'a suitable way' for him in revealing the nature of his disease. Suppose we attempt to find suitable clothes for someone, we can ask her favourite colour or design etc. or we can go and change them if she does not like what we chose for her. In the case of revealing a diagnosis, however, the patient cannot get involved in the process of finding the best way of telling her the truth, and the effect is irreversible if the 'suitable way' defined by the doctor is not really suitable for the patient. So the idea of 'finding a suitable way for each patient' is based upon the Japanese doctor's attitude that 'I know the patient better than he does himself', which takes the doctor's paternalism for granted. We do not intend to say that the disclosure of the diagnosis of incurable diseases will necessarily be done in an insensitive manner without choosing a suitable way of communication, but most Japanese doctors are not competent to understand the psychology of patients because they have not been 'trained' and educated to be good communicators with dying patients in their cure-centred and science biased medical education.

So there is a danger in discussing the issue of the disclosure of the diagnosis from the aspect of whether the doctor can find a most appropriate way for the patient's personality or mental state. There are at least two reasons for this. Firstly, most Japanese doctors are not capable of dealing with psychological aspects of patient care due to their lack of education; secondly, logically the patient cannot take part in finding the best way of telling the truth, since the patient's involvement in the search is impossible without his already knowing the truth.

As to 'the right not to know', Hoshino suggests that patients with all different kinds of diseases should fill in questionnaires at reception on their first visit to the hospital asking them in advance about their wishes concerning the diagnosis. Hoshino's suggestion is that if the patient indicates on this questionnaire that he or she does not want to know the diagnosis in the case of incurable disease, the diagnosis should not be told so that the patient's right not to know the truth is protected (Hoshino, 1991, pp.104-12). However, the problem is that there is no way in which the patient himself or herself can make sure if his or her 'right not to know' is preserved, because he or she cannot know it without knowing the truth, and also that the doctor still has to talk to the patient about his or her condition even though this may involve lying. Suppose the doctor conceals the diagnosis of advanced stomach cancer from a patient and instead says that she has a stomach ulcer, since it is her own wish that the truth is to be hidden. Because she does not know that her right 'not to know' will be protected, she may begin to become sceptical about her doctor's veracity when he gives her various painful treatments (for cancer) without her condition getting any better.

The difficulty is that she cannot take part in the process of respecting her right 'not to know'. At the point where the patient's right of this kind is respected, the patient cannot avoid being almost completely passive in the whole medical process and his or her autonomy cannot be respected because he or she cannot be autonomous without knowing the truth. There is another problem that the patient will inevitably be suspicious whenever the doctor tells her she has nothing serious even if it is the truth. The notion of the 'right not to know' does not therefore sit comfortably alongside other rights of the patient in medical decision-making. So, it is hard to protect both the 'right to know' and 'right not to know' without having the patient involved in the process of protecting those rights. The patient's involvement and awareness of the protection of his right is logically impossible in the latter case, as we have already explained.

This problem of 'truth telling' is one of the biggest obstacles to bringing the Western hospice movement to Japanese incurable cancer patients. The process of stopping concealing the diagnosis may be inevitable, if Japanese medicine really intends to spread hospice care whether inside or outside hospitals. This is not only because the Japanese patient cannot be a 'pilgrim' without knowledge of his or her disease, but also because hospice care cannot be popularized without letting the public know what a 'hospice' is meant to be. If Japan attempts to establish more hospice wards inside hospitals or hospice buildings independent from hospitals, it will be necessary to let people know that the hospice is for those who have got incurable diseases. Even if the term 'hospice' is dropped in favour of 'palliative care units', it will still not be easy to increase them without thinking about the disclosure of the diagnosis. This is because both 'hospices' and 'palliative care units' gather incurable cancer patients into one place, whether as part of a hospital building or in an independent building outside the hospital. They have to explain what sort of patients are concentrated in this one spot in order to increase public awareness of the need for 'hospice' or 'palliative care' and to gain support from charitable giving. When the public has knowledge of what 'hospice' or 'palliative care' is, patients will inevitably recognise themselves as having incurable cancer at the point that they are admitted.

One of the important things to be done in the present situation in Japan is to identify the question of from what aspect the disclosure of the truth should be considered: (i) from the aspect of good or bad consequences for the doctor? the patient? the family? some or all of them?; and (ii) from the point of view of individual rights no matter what the consequences are?; (iii) from both (i) and (ii)? The matter of whether the problem of 'truth telling' is considered from the question of 'consequences' or 'individual rights' will influence whether or not the truth is to be told to the patient and who the final decision-maker should be. In the current situation it is more likely that Japan will tend to consider the issue with respect to 1). This will make Japanese doctors hesitate to reveal the true nature of the disease to the patient while they are waiting for the perfect time to disclose the diagnosis, which will bring good consequences for everyone.

Japanese medical ethicists often speak as though the issue is not a matter of 'to tell or not to tell' but 'how, when, and what to tell, or who will tell'. The basic attitude found here is that the truth must not be told before the best conditions with regard to 'how', 'when', 'what', and 'who' have been met. In other words, the patient is entitled to the 'right to know the truth' only when the surrounding conditions match this standard. So the patient's right to know the diagnosis is not something which he or she possesses but something to be given externally normally by the doctor. But if the issue were thought of from an individual rights point of view, it would not be a matter of meeting requirements.

The tendency for important decisions in an individual's life to be made by others has been taken for granted in Japanese history. Perhaps this has been considered the best way of harmonising human relationships in Japanese society. In the case of 'truth telling', the doctor and the family may hide the truth through good intentions by considering the benefits to the patient, but they may also consider certain benefits for themselves to maintain the harmony of human relationships in the community, as can be found in the Japanese difficulty in accepting another person's death. Apart from loving and caring for a member of their community, it seems that the Japanese people make decisions for the person in order to benefit not only the person but also the whole community. We can call it, in a sense, a consequentialist morality, though it must be distinguished from Western consequentialism in so far as Western consequentialists try to respect the individuality of humans.

If the concept of hospice care cannot be popularized without the disclosure of the true diagnosis, Japan may need to look at the moral issues from a deontological point of view. Even if the consequence of hiding the diagnosis benefits everyone, the action itself may be morally wrong. This moral perspective has been forgotten by the Japanese in regard to this issue. If we consider the issue from the aspect of individual rights, we may suggest that the doctor should tell the diagnosis to the patient even if it might bring bad consequences and so he should try to prevent the predicted bad effects by using different strategies than just hiding the diagnosis. We doubt that 'truth telling' can become prevalent in the current 'consequentialist' way of thinking in Japan, where the interest lies mainly in 'how and when it is told', 'what is told', and 'who should tell' and there is no active concern to tell the truth unless the patient's mental and physical conditions and his surrounding environment meet certain requirements (e.g., see Chapter 3).

Japan may have to change its whole culture if it is to look at the issue of 'truth telling' as an individual's right, because this changes the meaning of disease and death from an event of the group into that of one individual. As we have already mentioned this may be the beginning of the fear of death as well. It may not be realistic to imagine, however, that the Japanese perspective on death, disease, and self, which has not really been changed essentially in the past centuries could be transformed suddenly. So, the meaning of the disclosure of the true diagnosis is different between the West and Japan. One possibility is that the whole community may be able to share the incurable cancer diagnosis with the patient as an event of all the family as they have always done in the matter of death. In this way, important medical decisions may be still made with and by the patient's family, as has been so in the patient's past life. The patient does not have to be 'a pilgrim', and cannot be so at any cost because a communal way of understanding human relationships will continue even after the disclosure of the diagnosis, and the patient may not have to take as much responsibility for his disease as the Western patient does. Considering Japanese people's attitudes to their own deaths, patients may more easily and passively accept their destiny as something sad rather than frightening.

The Japanese incurable cancer patient would then no longer be a 'baby', since there would be room for him to make decisions about his life and death together with his family. He would no longer be totally blind or in a 'sleeping state' as to his physical condition. What we are proposing here is the prospect of telling him the diagnosis without privatizing the patient's death and disease, but retaining the traditional community sharing. This will not suddenly change the Japanese attitude to death and disease, but modify the doctor's perspective on his relationship with and responsibility for the patient, because the patient is not now a 'baby', who is completely passive and blind without knowing of his or her condition, even though he or she may still be dependent upon the doctor or the family in other respects. An interesting issue here is that the disclosure could encourage the traditional Japanese sharing of death, because it allows the patient and the family to talk openly about the patient's disease and death as an event of the whole family. Communication and discussion on the subject between the patient and the family may be increased as well as between the family and the doctor. This shows that, although it may be still strong, the doctor's authority to influence the patient's dying process from various aspects will be reduced, and the dynamics of the human relationships amongst the doctor, the patient, and the family will be more balanced than before. Japanese doctors may still remain paternalistic even if they begin to honestly tell the diagnosis to the patient, but the bond of trust between the patient and the family maintained by 'truth telling' (openness in their communication) can more easily be defended even if the paternalism might cause harm, particularly to the patient. While the Japanese hospice at the moment leaves the doctor's and the family's guilt 'unpurified' because of their telling lies to the patient about the diagnosis (Chapters 2 and 4), the disclosure will clear this guilt.

In the case of hiding the truth from the patient, however, the family has to tell lies to the patient and, as a result of this, inevitably becomes distant from the patient psychologically or even physically, and asks the doctor for instructions about the process of medical decision-making for the patient. This destroys the bond of trust between the patient and the family. So, communication between the doctor and the family tends to be emphasized more than that between the doctor and the patient or the family and the patient. It isolates the patient from honest and open human relationships, and this can reinforce the doctor's paternalism or power to control the patient as well as the family.

One big question is how to define the meaning of 'truth telling' for Japanese people, if it was to begin. The expression the 'right to know' obliges us to concentrate on individuals, and in this way the patient's responsibility for his disease and death is heavier by being removed from others. In the Japanese tradition, an individual's rights have been protected by his or her family or community, who are supposed to make important decisions about his or her life. There does not seem to be a clear distinction between an individual's rights and his family's rights, and there has not been an awareness of such a need to distinguish them from one another in Japan. The expression 'right to know' may have different nuances between the West and Japan, since the word 'right' has a stronger meaning in individualistic Western societies than in Japan, where individuals' rights are preserved in a mixture of the concepts of individual rights and a group's rights.

Having understood the Japanese confusion of definition and consciousness in relation to 'individuals' and 'the group', we presuppose that the disclosure of the diagnosis to the patient will not tend to ruin the Japanese traditional way of thinking in regard to their attitude to death and disease, because it will not just involve the issue of 'individual rights'. Knowing the nature of the disease will not privatize the death of individuals as it does in the West, which leads them to fear death. But, then, the idea of a 'hospice pilgrimage' in the West based upon an individual awareness of one's own death and responsibility for death and disease will not be applicable to Japanese incurable cancer patients, and the Japanese 'hospice' without the notion of an individual 'pilgrimage' and 'cross' can be no longer called a 'hospice' unequivocally in relation to the Western concept.

The Establishment of the Hospice Outside Hospitals in Terms of a Patient-Community Relationship We shall consider the establishment of the hospice outside hospitals in terms of a patient's relationship with a community under the following headings:

the patient community relationship;
the establishment of independent hospices in Japan without producing 'strangers';
the different nature of the patient-community relationship between the West and Japan;
financial problems in establishing independent hospices in Japan;
consideration of the doctor's vulnerability.

The patient-community relationship   The Western hospice has redefined the ethos of human relationships from that of the doctor-patient relationship into the patient-community relationship. The possibility of the patient-community relationship is in part deeply related to the informal nature of hospice care, which does not rely on technical medical knowledge. In this form of relationship, the doctor's paternalism is much reduced because everyone can be a carer. The vulnerability - pain and stress - of the carers is shared and cared for, and the healers' masks of the carers can be completed by their understanding of and caring for their own vulnerability, because only through this can they truly appreciate patients' pain. In Japanese hospices, however, this patient-community relationship may not be easily created because they are often set inside hospital buildings, and thus the nature of human relationships in the hospital setting tends to be reflected in the hospice. Establishing hospice buildings outside hospitals, as the West has done, may be one of the easiest methods of renewing the form of human relationships within the medical environment, so that the doctor's paternalism is reduced by dividing the responsibility for patients between different carers without there being too much concentration on the doctor.

But this isolation of the hospice building from the hospital in the Western hospice movement has itself created part of its problems as was discussed through 'the pilgrim-cancer patient metaphor' in Chapter 2. The difficulty is that incurable cancer patients become 'strangers' or 'pilgrims' in society and the care of the dying or talking about death can be done only within the 'greenhouse' called the 'hospice'. As we earlier emphasized, Japanese incurable cancer patients cannot become 'pilgrims' whether the diagnosis is told to them or not, but there may be a risk that they become 'strangers' isolated from society through the establishment of independent buildings especially for dying cancer patients. Let us discuss then the possibility of such a risk, as we would hesitate to suggest that Japan build hospice buildings outside hospitals if it created the problem of 'greenhouses' in a similar way as in the Western hospice.

The paradox found in the Western hospice movement is produced by the fact that the hospice ideals, such as an open attitude to death and bereavement, are not reflected in the attitudes of people outside hospice care although they give financial support for building hospices. Incurable cancer patients become 'pilgrims' or 'strangers' who can have 'strawberries' (hospice type care) only from 'greenhouses' called hospices because it always remains a 'cold December' outside 'greenhouses'. The cause of this 'cold December' is that outside hospice care the public do not accept the hospice perspective of treating death and related emotional concerns as part of their lives, no matter how much they support the hospice movement and its philosophy.

The establishment of independent hospices in Japan without producing 'strangers' But if Japan developed hospice buildings outside hospitals, the situation might be different from in the West because outside hospices or hospitals it has not been a 'cold December' in Japan. The situation in Western hospitals tends to reveal the modern Western attitude to death and emotions, with these subjects being likely to be taboo both inside and outside hospitals. To a great extent, the current hospital's position in relation to the care of the dying and the tendency to dehumanize the treatment of such patients are reflections of a more general attitude to death and emotions in the West. The Western hospice movement (in an attempt to provide 'greenhouses' to grow 'strawberries') has developed on the whole as a reaction against these modern attitudes to death, dying, and emotions, as the Western world has become a 'wasteland'.

But, in Japan, the topic of death and emotions have not yet become taboo as much as in the West even in the modern period of urbanization and westernization, because of its communal sharing of these matters, so the public attitude to death is, in a way, opposite to the situation inside hospitals. The 'wasteland' for the Japanese is in fact mainly inside medicine and hospitals, and outside the hospital is not yet totally a 'cold December'. Even if Japan created hospices separately from hospital buildings, they might not be connected with an image like 'greenhouses' and might not produce a huge gap between the public attitude to death and its attendant emotions and what is going on inside hospices, so hospices which are independent from hospitals are not likely to produce 'strangers'. Thus, Japanese independent hospices may be able to mirror the Japanese traditional sharing of the events of death and related emotions, which has still remained in modern Japanese society. Considering that people's attitudes to death inside and outside the hospice are likely to be consistent in Japan, while they are inconsistent with each other in the West, establishing independent hospices in Japan may be stronger in influencing hospitals than in the West. It may be even easier for Japan to build independent hospice buildings than it has been for the West in this regard, since the Japanese hospice has to fight only against the dominant scientific culture of modern medicine but not the general public attitude to death and dying, while the Western hospice has to fight against both. Additionally, the establishment of independent hospices could overcome a negative impression which people may have towards the hospice because it is inside the hospital which is itself considered to be a 'dirty' place called 'byo-in' (a house of illness).

The different nature of the patient-community relationship between the West and Japan The differences which have been identified between the Western and Japanese situations may be a strength, if Japan can develop its services outside the hospital setting in order to find a quicker way of changing the nature of medical relationships from a doctor-centred one into a patient-community relationship. What is meant by the patient-community relationship in Japan may, however, be different from the Western one, because the patient is more passive and has less awareness of self or individual rights than the Western patient. It is likely that the Japanese doctor's position will remain superior to that of other carers even in the hospice outside the hospital. This is because the Japanese hospice movement began from inside the hospital while the first modern Western hospice was opened outside the hospital. So the Western hospice can bring a new definition of human relationships and each carer's role from the beginning. But, because the Japanese hospice movement began from inside the hospital, it cannot avoid modelling itself on the style of the hospital including that of human relationships. Even if hospices began to be instituted outside hospitals, they would be likely to try at the beginning to follow the old hospital patterns of the first ones. So the doctor's position may remain superior in the Japanese hospice even outside the hospital building. Nevertheless the patient-community relationship will make a big improvement in the attention given to the doctor's vulnerability together with that of other carers.

Financial problems in establishing independent hospices in Japan By the establishment of hospices outside hospitals, it may be possible to reconstruct human relationships in the medical environment so that the doctor and other carers can share their pain and stress. But this will not be easy without dealing with the serious financial problems involved in creating independent hospice buildings. One key to solving this problem might be hidden in the problem of 'truth telling', which is deeply related to the possibility of whether or not Japan can expand the hospice movement, as we explored earlier. If the hospice movement was known by more people in Japan, mass communication would begin to influence charitable fund raising. Hence there are interesting links between the disclosure of the diagnosis, the establishment of hospices independently from hospitals, and the overcoming of financial difficulties.

Consideration of the doctor's vulnerability We explored in Chapter 9 the traditional notion in Japanese medicine of 'Jin-jutsu' (the art of love and compassion) and that 'compassion' for the patient's pain and suffering requires the doctor to understand his own pain and suffering. As in the idea of the wounded healer in relation to the Western doctor, we may think about reviving the idea of an art of love and compassion in order to complete the doctor's healer's mask, since the Japanese doctor cannot help looking at his own vulnerability together with that of his patient if he truly tries to practise the art of love and compassion. As already explained in Chapter 4, the Japanese word for 'compassion' is 'do-jo', the characters for which mean the same flow of emotions, and the doctor needs to accept himself as having the same flow of emotions as that of his patients, such as sadness, anger, anxiety, fear, and so on, in order to feel compassion for his patients. Indeed the doctor needs to have a rich experience of all these emotions so that he can imagine what it is like when his patients feel each of them.

Thus we cannot solve the problem of the doctor-patient relationship without considering it from the angle of the doctor's vulnerability. However the doctor's vulnerability is neglected both in the West and Japan, and the doctor's paternalism is considered to be caused partly by his psychological defence in relation to his patients, through which he attempts to compensate for his unacknowledged vulnerability. Both Western and Japanese doctors are educated to be 'scientists', who treat diseases rather than persons, and they are not sufficiently educated in communication skills and psychology to deal with dying patients and do not get any significant support for their own psychological stress in medical practice. They are not allowed to be emotional even when facing traumatic events such as their patients' deaths or the families' bereavement because such emotions are considered to be a barrier to scientific objectivity. This situation encourages the doctor to be psychologically defensive and have an over-objective or distant attitude to his patients, and eventually leads him to inhuman as well as insensitive ways in treating his patients' pain and emotions. The doctor's healer's mask can never be completed without consideration of his vulnerability, and the revival of the idea of the 'wounded healer' in the West and 'jin-justu' (the art of love and compassion) in Japan will help the doctor to reduce his stress and pain.

The vulnerability of the Japanese doctor is more complex in nature than that of the Western doctor because the Japanese doctor suffers from a gap between his scientific attitude to the patient and his traditional Japanese attitudes especially in connection with death, dying and disease. Finding a good balance between the two is an important agenda for modern Japanese doctors, and the revival of medicine as 'jin-justu' (the art of love and compassion), which is concerned with the patients' pain through feeling and accepting the same flow of emotions within the doctors themselves, may help them to reach this balance. The redefinition of human relationships, as mentioned earlier, will reduce the stress and pain of the doctor by avoiding a concentration of medical responsibility for the patient on him alone and dividing it among all the carers, so sharing the stress and pain of the carers on a communal level. This is very close to the traditional Japanese way of treating death and its related emotions, so may help the Japanese doctor to fill the gap between his scientific and Japanese attitudes. In order to change the nature of human relationships in the Japanese hospital or hospice inside the hospital, it will be helpful to establish hospices independently from hospitals, as we mentioned earlier. The disclosure of the diagnosis is also very important, since it enables a public awareness and understanding of the concept of the hospice as independent from that of the hospital, and it can also reduce the doctor's responsibility for making decisions on the patient's behalf and the stress of telling lies to the patient.

Should 'It' be Called a 'Hospice'?

If the idea of individual responsibility for disease and death is necessary for the hospice philosophy, the Japanese hospice cannot be properly called a 'hospice', and this problem seems to be caused by the Japanese lack of understanding and an unclear definition of the principles that go to make up a 'hospice'. As an example, if Japan truly understood the Western hospice philosophy which implies the idea of 'an individual pilgrimage and a cross' and intended to follow this route itself, it could not help beginning a new policy of telling the truth about the disease to the patient. What Japan is doing in the name of hospice care is of course like hospice care in the West to a certain degree, particularly in its emphasis on the care of physical and psychological pain, but the perspective on death, dying, and the individual which is embedded in the Western hospice at a deep level, is different from that of the Japanese 'hospice' in the various senses that we have discussed. It is dangerous to bring to Japan only superficial elements of what is going on in the Western hospice and using the term 'hospice' regardless of the difference, since this may weaken the strength deriving from Japanese culture, such as the sharing of death and its attendant emotions and the relative lack of fear in relation to death. So it is advisable that the Japanese should first clarify what they are aiming for in the care of incurable cancer patients or the dying in general, and obtain a deeper understanding of what is meant by 'hospice care' in the West, so that they may use the term 'hospice care' with better discrimination or give such care a new name.

A Perspective on Home Care Nursing in Japanese Palliative Care

Considering the sympathetic relationship between the hospice perspective and the Japanese public attitude to death, we might consider the possibility of home care as another alternative. In the West, changing the nature of the care of dying cancer patients began first with the hospice movement establishing new institutions with a new philosophy of care and independent from hospitals. But the interest in Western terminal care is now moving towards home care nursing, which has been developed as one branch of the hospice movement (Taylor, 1983, p.9; cited by Clark, 1991, p.997). While the hospice has educated health care professionals in treating dying cancer patients particularly in the field of pain control, the nature of hospital care in relation to the dying is beginning to be influenced by hospice care as well (Seale, 1989, pp.551-59).

Japan may also be able to consider home care for terminal cancer patients in the community more easily than in the West, because of the Japanese traditional emphasis on the community sharing of death and dying as of all events of individuals' lives. In order to put this into practice, there are many hurdles to be jumped over in the current situation in Japan. Firstly, it will be necessary to change the nature of human relationships in health care such as the doctor-centred emphasis. This is because the idea of home care would be difficult to implement successfully without a change in the balance of power between the informal carers, who will mainly be patients' families, and the health care professionals. Otherwise, Japanese patients' families will tend to remain passive in front of the doctors and allow them unrestrained authority in the processes of medical decision-making. Also, the role of nurses would be very important in home care, where they are often expected to take the initiative, but the low status of Japanese nurses may not allow them to develop such a leading position. Moreover, the Japanese lay people's image of terminal cancer patients would need to be modified from that of 'those who only specialists can handle' into 'those who can be a focus for a team of caring staff and the family', through a deep understanding of symptom control and this can only be achieved with professional support to help them to gain this understanding.

Although the Japanese culture accords great respect to the community and the family sharing of death and dying which would be a great strength in developing home care for terminal cancer patients, the problems concerning the nature of human relationships in health care and the lay public's lack of confidence in their abilities to care for dying cancer patients in their community could not be solved immediately. It seems that Japan needs to have a 'testing period' during which it attempts to gradually change the situation allowing time to cope with the new relationships and attitudes, and independently established hospices may give health care professionals and families space to do so. Even if Japan built hospice buildings separately from hospitals, they would not become 'greenhouses' with the outside remaining a 'cold December' as in the West, and that means their existence would not easily become an obstacle to developing home care but might provide a strong base from which to support it.

However there is still a risk of the public's dependency upon the hospice in the case of establishing independent hospice buildings, and this might prevent them from taking the idea of home care seriously. Taking all these consideration into account, our recommendation for home care is, therefore, to develop hospices independently from hospitals together with home care systems, with a strong awareness of the need for home care as one of the main parts of hospice care before focusing too much on producing in-patient hospice care buildings. In the end, the ideal is that hospice buildings become instruments of home care, and home care becomes what the buildings are for. It should be possible to develop home care more quickly in Japan than in the West, once Japan succeeds in spreading the new notion of human relationships in medicine and in changing public awareness about terminal cancer, since there is not a 'greenhouse-wasteland problem' in Japan and the culture is already more in tune with the idea of home care.

Bibliography

Anesaki, M. (1930), *History of Japanese Religion with Special Reference to the Social and Moral Life of the Nation*, London, Kegan Paul, Trench, Trubrer & Co.

Anzai, T. and Okuse, T. (1981), *Rinshobamen ni okeru shinrigaku (Psychology in Clinical Medical Practice)*, Tokyo, Igakushoin.

Aries, P. (1974), *Western Attitude to Death from the Middle Ages to the Present*, London, John's Hopkins University Press.

Aries, P. (1981), *The Hour of Our Death*, London, Penguin Books Ltd.

Armstrong, R.C., (1950), *An Introduction to Japanese Buddhist Sect*, published by the author.

Baumeister, R. (1986), *Identity: Cultural Change and the Struggle for Self*, New York, Oxford University Press.

Becker, C. (1989), 'Buddhist Ethics for the New Century - Suicide and Euthanasia' *The Journal of Pure Land Buddhism* 6, pp.156-57.

Becker, C. (1992), 'Nihon no noushi-hantei-saiyou ni hantai suru riyu' (Why Japan Should Not Accept Brain Death Criteria), in Umehara, T. (ed.), *Noushi to Zouki Ishoku (Brain Death and Organ Transplants)*, Tokyo, Asahi Shinbun-sha, pp.237-65.

Becker, C., (1994), personal communication, 24th February.

Beloff, J. (1993a), 'Killing or Letting Die? Is there a valid moral distinction?' *News Letter of the Voluntary Euthanasia Society of Scotland* January.

Beloff, J. (1993b), personal communication.

Bennet, G. (1987), *The Wound and the Doctor Healing, Technology, and Power in Modern Medicine*, London. Secker & Warburg.

Carlin, M. (1989), 'Medieval English Hospitals', in Granshaw, L. and Porter, R. (eds), *The Hospital in History*, London, Routledge, pp.21-39.

Carlisle, J. (1992), 'Terminal Care Limited for AIDS', *Nursing Times* 88(15), p.7.

Cassell, E.J. (1978), *The Healer's Art*, New York, Penguin Books Ltd.

Cassell, E.J. (1991), *The Nature of Suffering and the Goals of Medicine*, Oxford, Oxford University Press.

Caudill, W. (1976), 'The Cultural and Interpersonal Context of Everyday Health and Illness in Japan and America', in Leslie, C. (ed.), *Asian Medical Systems*, Berkeley, University of California Press, pp.159-177.

Clark, D. (1991), 'Contradiction in the Development of New Hospices - A Case

Study', *Social Science and Medicine* 33(9), pp.995-1004

Clark, D. (1993), 'Whither the Hospices?' in Clark, D. (ed.) *The Future for Palliative Care Issues of Policy and Practice*, Buckingham, Philadelphia, Open University Press, pp.167-177.

Deken, A. (ed.) (1986a), *Shi wo kangaeru (Thinking of death)*, Tokyo, Medical Friend Ltd.

Deken, A. (ed.) (1986b), *Shi wo mitoru (Watching death)*, Tokyo, Medical Friend Ltd.

Department of Health and Social Security (DHSS) (1979), *Doctor/Patient Relationship A Study in General Practice*, London, Her Majesty's Stationary Office.

Dunstan, G. *et al.* (eds) (1972), *The Problem of Euthanasia*, Documentation in Medical Ethics.

Ekiken, K. (1711), *Kadokun (Introduction to a family way of life)*.

Endo, S. (ed.) (1992), *Anata ga Yamai ni Taoretara (When you become ill)*, Tokyo, Kyoto, PHP Kenkyu-jo.

Enmaru, T. (1978), *Shi no bunka-shi (A cultural history of death)*, Tokyo, Tairyu-sha Ltd.

An Etymological Dictionary of the English Language (1881), Oxford, Clarendon Press.

Fainsinger, R., *et.al.* (1991), 'Symptom Control During the Last Week of Life on a Palliative Care Unit', *Journal of Palliative Care* 7(1), pp.5-11.

Faulkner, A. (1993), 'Development in Bereavement Services', in Clark, D. (ed.), *The Future for Palliative Care Issues of Policy and Practice*, Buckingham, Philadelphia, Open University Press, pp.68-79.

Fisher, S. and Todd, A.D. (eds) (1983), *The Social Organization of Doctor-Patient Communication*, Washington D.C., Centre for Applied Linguistics.

Fromm, E. (1956), *The Art of Loving*, New York, Harper Bros.

Fulton, R. (1981), 'Hospice in America From Principle to Practice', in Saunders, C., Summers, D.H. and Teller, Neville (eds), *Hospice The Living Idea*, London, Edward Arnold, pp.9-18.

Furukawa, T. (1986), *Shi wa sukueruka - Iryo to shukyo no genten (Can we save death - the origin of medicine and religion)*, Tokyo, Chiyusha.

Fuse, S. (1969), *Ishi no rekishi - sono nihonteki tokucho (A history of doctoring - its Japanese nature)*, Tokyo, Chuko Shinsho.

Glover, J. (1990), *Causing Death and Saving Lives*, London, Penguin Books Ltd.

Gorer, G. (1964), *Shi to kanashimino shakaigaku (Death, grief, and mourning in contemporary Britain)* (translated by Utsunomiya, T), Tokyo, Yorudan Sha Ltd.

Groddeck, G.W. (1963), *Le livre du ça* Paris, Gallimard.

Granshaw, L. and Porter, R. (eds) (1989), *The Hospital in History*, London, Routledge.

Hara, Y. (1982), 'Nihonteki hospice no arikata' (The way of the Japanese

Hospice), in Ikemi, Y. and Nagata, K. (eds), *Shi no rinsho - Wagakuni ni okeru makki-kanja kea no jissai (The clinical aspect of death - Practice of the care of the terminally ill in Japan)*, Tokyo, Seishin Shobo, pp.103-117.

Henderson, J. (1989), 'The Hospitals of Late-Medieval and Renaissance Florence: A Preliminary Survey', in Granshaw, L. and Porter, R. (eds), *The Hospital in History*, London, Routledge, pp.63-92.

Herzlich, C. and Pierret, J. (1987), *Illness and Self in Society*, translated by Forster, E., Baltimore, The John's Hopkins University Press.

Hill, F. (1989), *An Examination of the Philosophical Foundation of the Modern Hospice Movement*, MA dissertation, Philosophy and Health Care, University of Wales.

Holy Bible King James Version.

Hoshino, K. (1991), *Iryo no rinri (Ethics of medicine)*, Tokyo, Iwanami shoten.

Humphrey, D. (1992), *Final Exit*, New York, A Dell Trade Paperback.

Ikemi, Y. (1982), 'Balint-hoshiki niyoru shi no rinsho no kyoiku' (The teaching of clinical thanatology by the Balint Method), in Ikemi, Y. and Nagata, K. (eds), *Shi no rinsho - Wagakuni ni okeru makki-kanja kea no jissai (The clinical aspect of death - practice of the care of the terminally ill in Japan)*, Tokyo, Seishin Shobo, pp.256-268.

Ikemi, Y. and Nagata, K. (eds) (1982), *Shi no rinsho - Wagakuni ni okeru makki-kanja kea no jissai (The clinical aspect of death - practice of the care of the terminally ill in Japan)*, Tokyo, Seishin Shobo.

Infield, G.B. (1974), *Disaster at Bari*, London, Hale.

Inoue, H. (1986), 'Gendai no nihonjin ni totteno shi' (Death for the Modern Japanese) in Deken, A. (ed.), *Shi wo kangaeru (Thinking of death)*, Tokyo: Medical Friend Ltd., pp.173-192.

Inoue, K. (1981), 'Gan kenkyukai fuzoku byoin de no toshokan sabisu' (Voluntary Work at the Library at the Hospital Attached to the National Institute of Cancer Research), *Byoin Toshokan* 3(2), pp.3-6.

Ishiwata, R. and Sakai, A. (1994), 'The Physician-Patient Relationship and Medical Ethics in Japan', *Cambridge Quarterly of Health Care Ethics* 3, pp.60-66.

James, N. and Field, D. (1992), 'The Routinization of Hospice: Charisma and Bureaucratization', *Social Science and Medicine* 34(12), pp.1363-1375.

Japan Society for Dying with Dignity (1992), *Newsletter*, Vol. 67.

Jung, C. (1954), *The Practice of Psychotherapy Collected Works Vol.16*, London: Routledge and Kegan Paul.

Kashiwagi, T. (1986), 'Hospice to iumono' (What is meant by 'hospice'), in Deken, A. (ed), *Shi wo mitoru (Watching death)*, Tokyo, Medical Friend Ltd., pp.229-54.

Kashiwagi, T. (1991a), 'Taminal kea to shomin no shi' (Terminal care and death of ordinary people), in Tada, T. and Kawai, H. (eds), *Sei to shi no yoshiki - Noishi jidai wo mukaeru nihon-jin no shisei-kan (The style of life and death -*

the Japanese attitude to death and life in the age of brain-death)*, Tokyo, Seishin Shobo, pp.83-96.

Kashiwagi, T. (1991b), 'Palliative Care in Japan', *Palliative Medicine* 5, pp.165-170.

Kashiwagi, T. (1993), 'Yodogawa kirisuto byoin hospice' (Yodogawa Christian Hospice), *The Japanese Journal of Hospice and Palliative Care*, 3(5), pp.363-68.

Kawai, H. (1991), 'Nihonjin no shisei-kan' (The Japanese attitude to death and life), in Tada, T. and Kawai, H. (eds), *Sei to shi no yoshiki - Noishi jidai wo mukaeru nihon-jin no shisei-kan (The style of life and death - the Japanese attitude to death and life in the age of brain-death)*, Tokyo, Seishin Shobo, pp.247-62.

Kawano, T. (1988), 'Bioethics and Terminal Care', *Thanatology* 1, Tokyo, Gijutsu Shuppan, pp.183-94.

Kearl, M.C. (1989), *Endings A Sociology of Death and Dying*, Oxford, Oxford University Press.

Kendall, A. (1970), *Medieval Pilgrims*, London, Wayland Publishers Ltd.

Kidel, M. (1988), 'Illness and Meaning', in Kidel, M. and Rowe-Leete, S. (eds), *The Meaning of Illness*, London, Routledge, pp.4-21.

King, G.G. (1920), *The Way of Saint James*, I, New York.

Kino, K. (1986), 'Bukkyo ni okeru shi to raiseikan' (The idea of death and the life after death in Buddhism), in Deken, A. (ed.), *Shi wo kangaeru (Thinking of death)*, Tokyo, Medical Friend Ltd., pp.130-49.

Knight, J.A. (1988), 'The Practice of Medicine', in Van Eys, J. and McGovern, J.P. (eds), *The Doctor as a Person*, Springfield, Illinois, Charles C. Thomas, pp.29-42.

Konishi, Y. (1991), 'A Perspective on Self-Decision Making' *The Japanese Journal of Clinical Research on Death and Dying* 18, p.465.

Kubler-Ross, E. (1969), *On Death and Dying*, London, Tavistock Publications.

Kubler-Ross, E. (1983), *On Children and Death (Shin Shinu Shunkan)*, translated by Akiyama, T. *et.al.*, Tokyo, Yomiuri Shinbun Sha.

Lipscomb, H. (1988), 'The Physician as the Bearer of Good or Bad News', in Van Eys, J. and McGovern, J.P. (eds), *The Doctor as a Person*, Springfield, Illinois, Charles C. Thomas, pp.93-110.

Maguire, P. (1985), 'Barriers to Psychological Care of the Dying', *British Medical Journal* 291, pp.1711-13.

Manning, M. (1984), *The Hospice Alternative - Living with Dying*, London, Souvenir Press.

Miller, R.J. (1992), 'Hospice Care as an Alternative to Euthanasia', *Law, Medicine and Health Care* 20, pp.I-2.

Minami, H. (1971), *Psychology of the Japanese People*, translated by Ikoma, A.R., Tokyo, University of Tokyo Press.

Mizuguchi, K., [with Takamiya, Y., Tanaka, K. and Ozaki, Y.] (1991), 'An

Investigation of The Terminal Care Education for Doctors Before and After Their Graduation' [discussion], in *The Japanese Journal of Terminal Care* 1(7), pp.472-78.

Mori, T. (1992), 'The Historical Medical World in Japan and Its Ideological Paradigm', *Annals of the Japanese Association for Philosophical and Ethical Researches in Medicine* 10, pp.25-45.

Morioka, M.(1989), *Brain-Dead Person*, Tokyo, Tokyo Shoseki.

Morris, C. (1972), *The Discovery of the Indivdiual 1050-1200*, London, S.P.C.K.

Mowat, L. (1993), 'Inconsistency' [poem], *VESS (the Voluntary Euthanasia Society for Scotland) Newsletter*

Munley, A. (1983), *The Hospice Alternative A New Context for Death and Dying*, New York, Basic Books Inc. Publishers.

Murphy, C.S. (1989), 'From Friedenheim to Hospice: A Century of Cancer Hospitals', in Granshaw, L. and Porter, R. (eds), *The Hospital in History*, London, Routledge, pp.221-241.

Murray, R.M. (1977), 'Psychiatric Illness in Male Doctors and Controls: An Analysis of Scottish Hospitals In-patient Data', *British Journal of Psychiatry*, 131, pp.1-10.

Nagao, R. and Yonemoto, S. (eds), *Meta-Bioethics: Seimei-kagaku to Houtetsugaku no taiwa (Meta-Bioethics: a dialogue of Life Science and Philosophy of Law)*, Tokyo, Nihon Hyoron Sha.

Nagata, K. (1982), 'Gan kokuchi no mondai (The problem of cancer diagnosis). In Ikemi, Y & Nagata, K.: *Shi no rinsho - Wagakuni ni okeru makki-kanja kea no jissai (The clinical aspect of death - practice of the care of the terminally ill in Japan)*, Tokyo, Seishin Shobo, pp.3-13.

Naito, I. (1992), 'Hospice no riso to kongo - Mazu nikutaiteki oyobi seishinteki kutsuu wo jokyo suru doryoku wo' (The hospice ideal and its future - making an effort to remove physical and psychological pain), in Endo, S. (ed), *Anata ga yamai ni taoretara (When you become ill)*, Tokyo, Kyoto, PHP Kenkyu-jo, pp.157-173.

Nakajima, Y. (1988), *Cultural History of Disease*, Tokyo, Yukankaku Shuppan.

Nara, M. (1987), 'Ronen no iryoto bukkyo-shiso - Shin-jidai no igaku-shiso wo motomete' (Health care for the elderly and Buddhist philosophy - the search for a philosophy of medicine for the new age), *Annals of the Japanese Association for Philosophical and Ethical Researches of Medicine* 5, pp.89-97.

Nichols, K.A. (1984), *Psychological Care in Physical Illness*, London, Chapman and Hall.

Nishikawa, K. (no date) Lecture for nurses.

Nishimura, K. (1991), 'Shiniyuku kodomo to shonikai' (Dying children and the paediatrician), *The Japanese Journal of Terminal Care*, 1(2), pp.91-95.

Nowwen, H.J.M. (1972), *The Wounded Healer*, New York, Doubleday.

Ohnuki-Tierney, E. (1984), *Illness and Culture in Contemporary Japan - an*

Anthropological View, Cambridge, Cambridge University Press.

Oki, T. (1991), *Songen aru shi (Death with dignity)*, Tokyo, Futami Shobou Ltd.

Ono, M. (1979), 'Kiko kokoro' (Listening heart), lecture given at Chiba University Hospital, 17th October.

Oxford Advanced Learners Dictionary (1989), Oxford, Oxford University Press.

The Oxford Dictionary of English Etymology (1966), Oxford, The Clarendon Press.

Pascal, B. (1946), *Prière pour le bon usage des maladies (Prayer for Making Good Use of Illness)*, Paris, Editions à l'Enfant Poète, p.110.

Philippi, D. (1959), *Norito A New Translation of the Ancient Japanese Ritual Prayers*, Tokyo, The Institute for Japanese Culture and Classics, Kokugakuin University.

Razan, H. (1629), *Shunkansho (Treatise on five virtues)*.

Registrar General (1978), England and Wales 1970-72, Occupational mortality, in *Decennial Supplement*, London, Her Majesty's Stationary Office.

Reich, W. (1975), *La Biopathie Du Cancer* Paris, Payot.

Sagara, R. (1984), *Nohonjin no shiseikan (The Japanese attitude to death and life)*, Tokyo, Perikan Sha Ltd.

Sakari, M. (1980), 'Gan-kanja ni Shinjitsu wo tsugemasuka?' (Do you tell the truth to cancer patients?)', *Nikkei Medical*, August, pp.48-52.

'Salute to the Hospice Movement' [Early Day Motion] (1992), *Notices of Motions*, 20 January, No.43, London, Her Majesty's Stationery Office, p.1571.

Sasaki, H. (1986), 'Minzoku no naka no shi (shi no minzoku)' (Death in folk customs (folk customs of death)), in Deken, A. (ed), *Shi wo kangaeru (Thinking of death)*, Tokyo, Medical Friend Ltd., pp.150-72.

Saunders, C. (1972), 'The Care of the Dying Patient and His Family', in Dunstan, G. *et al.* (eds), *The Problem of Euthanasia*, Documentation in Medical Ethics.

Saunders, C. (1977), *St Christopher's Hospice Annual Report 1976-1977*, London, St Christopher's Hospice.

Saunders, C. (1980), 'Euthanasia: Caring to the End', *Nursing Mirror*, 151(10), (September 4), pp.52-3.

Saunders, C., Summers, D.H. and Teller, Neville (eds) (1981), *Hospice The Living Idea*, London, Edward Arnold

Saunders, C. (1984), 'St Christopher's Hospice', in Shneidman, E. (ed.), *Death Current Perspectives*, 3rd edition, Alto, Mayfield Publishing, pp.266-71.

Saunders, E.D. (1964), *Buddhism in Japan With an Outline of Its Origins in India*, Westport, Connecticut, Greenwood Press.

Sawada, A. (1992) 'The Problem of the Shortage of Nursing Labor in Japan', (a paper presented at the 6th conference of the European Society for Philosophy of Medicine and Health Care, Budapest, 14th August)

Seale, C. (1989), 'What Happens in Hospices: A Review of Research', *Social*

Science and Medicine, 28, pp.551-59.

Seale, C. (1991a), 'Death from Cancer and Death from Other Causes: The Relevance of the Hospice Approach', *Palliative Medicine*, 5, pp.1-19.

Seale, C. (1991b), 'Communication and Awareness About Death - A Study of a Random Sample of Dying People', *Social Science and Medicine*, 32(8), pp.943-52.

Segawa, S. (1988), *The Actual Spot of Heart Transplant*, Tokyo, Shincho Sha.

Shaw, G.B. (1991), *Pygmalion*, Harlow, Longman Group U.K. Ltd.

Sherwin, S. (1992), *No Longer Patient   Feminist Ethics and Health Care*, Philadelphia, Temple University Press.

Shinjigen (dictionary of Chinese characters) (1969), Tokyo, Kadokawa Shoten, (first published 1968).

Shneidman, E.S. (ed.) (1984), *Death   Current Perspectives*, Alto, Mayfield Publishing

Shneidman, E.S. (1986), *Shiniyukutoki soshite nokosarerumono (Deaths of man)*, translated by Shirai, T. *et al.*. Tokyo, Seishin Shobou Ltd.

Shorter, E. (1985), *Bedside Manners: The Troubled History of Doctors and Patients*, New York, Simon and Shuster.

Snow, H. (1896), 'Opium and Cocaine in the Treatment of Cancerous Disease', *The British Medical Journal 2*, p.718.

Sontag, S. (1978), *Illness as Metaphor*, London, Penguin Books Ltd.

SPA! (1991), (Special issue on death) November 6th.

Stoddard, S. (1979), *The Hospice Movement*, London, Jonathan Cape.

Sullivan, J.V. (1950), *The Morality of Mercy Killing*, The Newman Press.

Tada, T. and Kawai, H. (eds) (1991), *Sei to shi no yoshiki - Noishi jidai wo mukaeru nihon-jin no shisei-kan (The style of life and death - The Japanese attitude to death and life in the age of brain-death)*, Tokyo, Seishin Shobo.

Takamiya, Y. (1991), 'Terminal care wa haiboku no igaku dewanai' (Terminal Care Is Not the Medicine of Defeat), *The Japanese Journal of Terminal Care*, 1(7), pp.468-471.

Talbot, C. (1967), *Medicine in Medieval England*, London, Oldbourne Books.

Taylor, H. (1983), *The Hospice Movement in Britain   Its Role and Its Future*, London, Centre for Policy on Ageing

The Terrence Higgins Trust and King's College, London (1992), *Living Will (explanatory notes and declaration form)*, London, The Terrence Higgins Trust and King's College, London.

Turner, B.S. (1987), *Medical Power and Social Knowledge*, London, Sage Publications.

Umehara, T. (ed.) (1992), *Noushi to Zouki Ishoku (Brain Death and Organ Transplants)*, Tokyo, Asahi Shinbun-sha.

Van Eys, J. and McGovern, J.P. (eds) (1988), *The Doctor as a Person*, Springfield, Illinois, Charles C. Thomas.

Vaux, K.L. (1988) 'The Physician as Priest', in Van Eys, J. and McGovern, J.P.

(eds), *The Doctor as a Person*, Springfield, Illinois, Charles C. Thomas, pp.127-134.

Veatch, R. (1991), *The Patient-Physician Relation*, Bloomington, Indiana University Press.

Ventafridda, V. (1990), 'Symptom Prevalence and Control During Cancer Patients' Last Days of Life', *Journal of Palliative Care* 6(3), pp.7-11.

Wallen, J., Waitzkin, H.B. and Stoeckle, J.D. (1979), 'Physicians' Stereotypes about Female Health and Illness: A Study of Patient's Sex and the Informative Process During Medical Interviews', *Women and Health* 4, pp.135-146.

Watanabe, T. (1988), *Shigaku - Alternative Lifestyle Catalogue*, Tokyo, Niki Shuppan.

West, C. (1983), '"Ask Me No Questions ... ' An Analysis of Queries and Replies in Physician-Patient Dialogues', in Fisher, S. and Todd, A.D. (eds), *The Social Organization of Doctor-Patient Communication*, Washington, D.C., Centre for Applied Linguistics, pp.75-106.

Wilson, J.B. (1975), *Death by Decision: The Medical Moral, and Legal Dilemmas of Euthanasia*, Philadelphia, The Westminster Press.

Yamamoto, Z., Sakamoto. T. and Takahashi, M. (1990), 'Do Terminal Patients Find Religious Support Necessary?', *Annals of the Japanese Association for Philosophical and Ethical Researches in Medicine* 8, pp.25-34.

Yamazaki, A. (1992), 'Yutakana sei to yasurakana shi' (An abundant life and a peaceful death), in Endo, S. (ed.), *Anata ga Yamai ni Taoretara (When you become ill)*, Tokyo, Kyoto, PHP Kenkyu-jo, pp.136-7.

Yamazaki, A. (1993), 'Sei Yohane Kai Sakuramachi Boyoin, Sei Yohane Hospice' (St John's Hospice in St John's Sakuramachi Hospital), *Japanese Journal of Hospice and Palliative Care*, 3(5), pp.358-62.

Yanagida, K. (1986), *Shi no Igaku Josho (An Introduction of Medicine of Death)*. Tokyo, Shincho Sha.

Yonemoto, S. (1987), 'Seimei-kagaku no tachiba kara' (From a viewpoint of Life Science), in Nagao, R. and Yonemoto, S. (eds), *Meta-Bioethics: Seimei-kagaku to Hou-tetsugaku no taiwa (Meta-Bioethics: a dialogue of Life Science and Philosophy of Law)*, Tokyo, Nihon Hyoron Sha, pp.217-226.

Index

Words used principally metaphorically are in single inverted commas.